S0-ECN-778

RELATED SERVICES FOR HANDICAPPED CHILDREN

RELATED SERVICES FOR HANDICAPPED CHILDREN

Edited by

`A15022 476844`

Morton M. Esterson, M.Ed., C.A.S.E.
Adjunct Professor of Special Education
Department of Education
Loyola College
Baltimore, Maryland

Linda F. Bluth, Ed.D.
Coordinator, Office of Nonpublic Placements
Baltimore City Public Schools
Baltimore, Maryland

HV
888.5
.R45
1987
west

ASU WEST LIBRARY

A College-Hill Publication
Little, Brown and Company
Boston/Toronto/San Diego

College-Hill Press
A Division of Little, Brown and Company (Inc.)
34 Beacon Street
Boston, Massachusetts 02108

© 1987 by Little, Brown and Company (Inc.)

All rights, including that of translation, reserved. No part of this publication may be reproduced, stored in a retrieval system, or transmitted in any form or by any means, electronic, mechanical, recording, or otherwise, without the prior written permission of the publisher.

Library of Congress Cataloging-in-Publication Data

Related services for handicapped children.

    Bibliography: p. 145.
    Includes index.
    1. Handicapped children—Services for—United States.
2. Handicapped children—Education—United States.
I. Esterson, Morton M., 1926–   . II. Bluth, Linda F.,
1943–   . [DNLM: 1. Child, Exceptional.
2. Handicapped. 3. School Health Services. 4. Social Work. WA 350 R382]
HV888.5.R45 1986 362.4′048′088054 86-14804.

ISBN 0-316-10045-5

Printed in the United States of America

CONTENTS

PREFACE

This timely book has been written for the school administrator, general educator, special educator, therapist, advocate, parent, and others interested in special education and related services provided to handicapped children. It examines the related service provisions as they currently relate to special education, and presents a clear understanding of the relationship between special education and related services. It familiarizes the reader with Public Law 94-142, The Education For All Handicapped Children Act of 1975; Public Law 98-199, The Education of the Handicapped Act Amendments of 1983; and the related services as defined in the law and its regulations.

Each chapter has been written by an experienced practitioner, who describes the various facets of related services on the basis of his or her professional training and personal experience. Controversial issues such as clean intermittent catheterization (CIC) and other health-related questions are thoroughly discussed. Throughout the book, an attempt is made to increase and facilitate an awareness of the impact of related service provisions upon special education.

Notes to the Reader: The words 'child' and 'children' as used in this text refer, in all cases, to the learner.

In Part II, 'Related Services,' the services are dealt with in alphabetical order, just as they are in PL94-142.

LIST OF CONTRIBUTORS

Shiela Applestein, M.S., CCC/SP
Speech-Language Pathologist
Baltimore City Public Schools
Baltimore, Maryland

Grace Black, R.N., M.S.N.
Community Health Nursing
  Supervisor
Baltimore City Health Department
Baltimore, Maryland

Thelma L. Blumberg, M.S.
School Psychologist
Baltimore City Public Schools
Baltimore, Maryland

Linda F. Bluth, Ed.D.
Coordinator, Office of Nonpublic
  Placements
Baltimore City Public Schools
Baltimore, Maryland

Thomas V. Dorsett, M.D., M.P.H.
Medical Director, Children and
  Youth Project
Baltimore City Health Department
Baltimore, Maryland

Morton M. Esterson, M.Ed.,
  C.A.S.E.
Adjunct Professor of Special
  Education
Department of Education
Loyola College
Baltimore, Maryland

Samuel H. Esterson, M.A., P.T.
Vice President
Capital Rehabilitation, Inc.
Baltimore, Maryland

Charlotte Exner, M.S., O.T.R.
Assistant Professor
Department of Occupational
  Therapy
Towson State University
Towson, Maryland

Brad Friedrich, Ph.D.
Chief of Audiology
Department of Communication
  Sciences and Disorders
The Kennedy Institute for
  Handicapped Children
Baltimore, Maryland

Janie R. Friedlander, M.S., C.A.S.
School Psychologist
Baltimore City Public Schools
Baltimore, Maryland

Lois Therres Pommer, Ed.D.
Clinical Supervisor/School
  Psychologist
The Kennedy Institute for
  Handicapped Children
Baltimore, Maryland

Maryanne Conlon Ralls, M.Ed.
Educational Specialist
Office of Nonpublic Placements
Baltimore City Public Schools
Baltimore, Maryland

Stuart M. Tabb, Ph.D., L.C.S.W.
Court Consultant
Baltimore City Public Schools
Baltimore, Maryland

Dennis Whitehouse, M.D.,
    M.R.C.P., F.A.A.P.
Associate Professor of Pediatrics
Johns Hopkins University
Director of Diagnostic and
    Evaluation Center
The Kennedy Institute for
    Handicapped Children
Baltimore, Maryland

PART I
BACKGROUND

Chapter 1

Introduction

Morton M. Esterson

The general philosophy of public school systems in the early twentieth century was to enroll handicapped children in either regular education classes, in special education classes, or in special schools. This prevailing philosophy continued until 1954, when the United States Supreme Court in the case of *Brown* v. *Topeka Board of Education* decided that state laws that permitted or required segregation of public schools violated the equal protection clause of the Fourteenth Amendment of the United States Constitution. Segregated or separate education was declared inherently unequal.

This ruling, together with research studies that indicated that handicapped children assigned to regular grades make greater academic gains than handicapped children placed in separate classes, encouraged and motivated parents of handicapped children to bring legal action against school systems. These suits resulted in rulings that all handicapped children have an inherent right to a free, appropriate public education (*Pennsylvania Association for Retarded Citizens v. Commonwealth of Pennsylvania*, 1971; *Mills v. Board of Education of the District of Columbia*, 1972; *Maryland Association for Retarded Citizens v. Baltimore City, Baltimore County, Montgomery County, Prince Georges County, and Maryland State Department of Education*, 1973; *Le Banks v. Spears*, 1975). It was this type of prominent litigation that resulted in adoption by almost every state of special legislation regarding the education of handicapped children (Turnbull and Schultz, 1979). Today, the majority of special education programs are a direct result of organized advocacy efforts, legislative campaigns, and litigation.

According to Wallace (1980), congressional findings as of 1975 revealed that there were more than 8 million handicapped children in the

United States and that the special education needs of many handicapped children were not being met. More than one half of all handicapped children were not receiving appropriate education services. One million handicapped children were excluded from public education. The climate was ripe for Congressional legislation in behalf of handicapped children.

On November 29, 1975, President Gerald R. Ford signed into law the Education for All Handicapped Children Act (EHA). This historic piece of legislation in behalf of all handicapped children is known as Public Law 94-142. Roberts and Hawk (1980) hold that PL 94-142 is, in reality, a civil rights law designed to present equal opportunities for a minority group, handicapped children. This federal civil rights legislation does not wrest educational authority from the states. With the passage of PL 94-142, each state assumed the legal responsibility for educating all handicapped children regardless of the nature or severity of their handicapping conditions. A lack of funding or resources may not be an excuse for noncompliance with the Education for All Handicapped Children Act.

WHICH CHILDREN ARE HANDICAPPED?

Public Law 94-142 defines handicapped children as those children who are mentally retarded, hard of hearing, deaf, speech-impaired, visually handicapped, seriously emotionally disturbed, orthopedically impaired, other health impaired, deaf-blind, multi-handicapped, or who have specific learning disabilities and who because of those impairments need special education and related services (Education of the Handicapped Regulations, 1985).

According to this definition, only those children who by reason of their handicap need special education and related services are considered handicapped. The law acknowledges that not every child with a handicapping condition will require special education and related services (Schifani, Anderson, and Odle, 1980).

WHAT IS SPECIAL EDUCATION?

The term special education, according to PL 94-142, means instruction specially designed, at no cost to the parent, to meet the unique needs of a handicapped child, including classroom instruction, instruction in physical education, home instruction, and instruction in hospitals and institutions (Education of the Handicapped Regulations, 1985).

A child in need of special education may also be entitled to receive related services if they are required to help the child benefit from special education.

WHAT ARE RELATED SERVICES?

Related services, as defined in PL 94-142, are transportation and such developmental, corrective, and other supportive services as are required to assist a handicapped child to benefit from special education; they include speech pathology and audiology, psychological services, physical and occupational therapy, recreation, early identification and assessment of disabilities in children, counseling services, and medical services for diagnostic or evaluative purposes. The term also includes school health services, social work services in schools, and parent counseling and training (Education for the Handicapped Regulations, 1985).

Obviously, not all related services will be required for each handicapped child. It is only when the service is required to assist a handicapped child to benefit from special education that it is covered under Public Law 94-142.

Since the implementation of PL 94-142, the related services provision has generated considerable controversy, because the listing of related services within the law is not exhaustive. Related services may include other developmental, corrective, and supportive services, such as art, music, artistic and cultural programs, and dance therapy, if they are required to assist a handicapped child to benefit from special education. It would also appear that any service, except for a medical service that is provided by a doctor and is not performed for diagnostic or evaluative purposes, that would enable a handicapped child to benefit from special education and is within reason to make the classroom physically accessible to him or her could be considered a related service (Rapp, 1985).

Currently, some 24 states have legislated related services requirements that are not specifically mentioned in the federal laws. Among these services are mobility training, summer school programs, special facilities, materials, and equipment.

An interesting example of the interpretation of the related services clause of PL 94-142 is the 1981 case of *Espino* v. *Besteiro*. This case presents an account of a child who was in an automobile accident and could no longer function in his classroom unless it was temperature controlled. The school district provided the child with a portable air-conditioned cubicle in which to work while in the classroom. The court, however, ruled that air-conditioning in this case was a related service necessary for the child to benefit from special education. It, therefore, ordered the school district to air condition the entire classroom so that the child could more fully interact with his teacher and with his classmates (Osborne, 1984; Piele, 1982).

Just as special education is to be provided at no cost to the parent, so too must related services be provided free, at no cost to the parent or guardian. Although the expense for providing related services may be high, the total cost for related services does not have to be paid entirely from education funds. Copayments may be made from other federal, state, local, and private sources. Title XIX medical funds, for example, may in some states be used to pay for related services. In other states, however, where the payment for health services is the total responsibility of the local education agency, Title XIX funds may not be used for related services (Shrybman, 1982).

The Education for All Handicapped Children Act requires every state, as well as the District of Columbia, American Samoa, Guam, the Trust Territory. of the Pacific Islands, the Commonwealth of Puerto Rico, the Northern Mariana Islands, and the Virgin Islands, to develop a clearly written policy that will assure every handicapped child the right to a free appropriate education at public expense. This educational program must include special education and related services. It is important to note that if a child does not require special education, no related services are required to be provided.

Each local education agency or school district, in compliance with its own state and local laws, is responsible for carefully considering each handicapped child's need for related services on a case-by-case basis and for making a reasonable determination as to whether a particular related service is needed to allow a child to benefit from special education. If a related service is not required to be provided during the school day, and can be provided other than during school hours, the local school district is not required to provide that service. If the related service, however, is necessary for the child to gain access to or benefit from special education, the school district must make provision for it at no cost to the parent.

When a school district or an Individualized Education Program (IEP) committee makes a decision that a handicapped child needs a related service, that service must be recorded on the child's Individualized Education Program. The extent and duration of the related service must be specified. This information will allow all members of the IEP committee to know the related service to be provided, and the number, the length, and the frequency of sessions during which the service is to be provided. The individual responsible for providing the related service will then be able to implement the service as indicated on the child's Individualized Education Program.

Basically, the courts have ruled that developmental, corrective, and supportive services of a nonmedical nature must be provided to a handicapped child if those services are needed for the child to make satisfactory progress toward the goals stated in his or her IEP. However, if a child is already benefitting from a special education program without the related service, the related service has not been required.

If there is a disagreement about whether a related service is necessary, the matter should be referred for a due process hearing. The due process procedure should be considered only after all attempts at negotiation or mediation have failed.

On December 2, 1983, President Ronald Reagan signed Public Law 98-199, the Education of the Handicapped Act Amendments of 1983. A requirement of the act is that the Secretary of the Department of Education must collect appropriate data concerning programs and projects supported by EHA from state and local educational agencies on at least an annual basis. The data to be collected shall include the following:

1. The number of handicapped children and youths receiving a free appropriate education and related services, by disability category and by age groups (3–5; 6–11; 12–17; and 18–21 years).
2. The amount of federal, state, and local funds each state expends for special education and related services.
3. The number and types of personnel employed for the provision of special education and related services to the handicapped children and youth, by disability category.
4. The estimated number and types of additional personnel, by disability category, needed to adequately carry out the policy established by PL 94-142.
5. A description of the special education and related services needed to fully implement PL 94-142 in each state, including estimates of the number of handicapped children and youth within each disability category and by age group (3–5; 6–11; 12–17; and 18–21 years) in need of improved services and of the types of programs and services in need of improvement.

In addition, PL 98-199 authorizes the Secretary to make preschool incentive grants to states that provide special education and related services to handicapped children from birth to 3 years of age (EHLR Special Report, 1984).

The Education for All Handicapped Children Act of 1975 and the Education of the Handicapped Act Amendments of 1983 mandate the provision of special education and related services for all handicapped children. The interpretation and implementation of these acts are the responsibility of each school district. The district may wish to provide in-service training for its personnel and related services providers to ensure consistency in the provision of required services. If there is a shortage of qualified personnel or an annual turnover of staff, modifications in the delivery of service models will be necessary. Different IEP teams may be required for different delivery models. The lack of funding and the unavailability of specialized equipment present a challenge to school districts to develop unique and innovative related services delivery systems. In the spirit and intent of PL 94-142 and PL 98-199, services to handicapped children should be considered on a case-by-case basis.

REFERENCES

Education of the Handicapped Regulations. (1985). 34 Code of Federal Regulations Part 300, Supplement 138.

EHLR Special Report: Amendments of EHA by PL 98-199, Supplement 112 (1984).

Espino v. Besteiro, 520 F. Supp. 905 (1981).

Osborne, A. G., Jr. (1984). How the courts have interpreted the related service mandate. *Exceptional Children, 51,* 249–252.

Piele, P. K. (1982). *Yearbook of school law* (pp. 132–133). Topeka, KS: National Organization on Legal Problems of Education.

Rapp, J. A. (1985). *Education law* (Vol. 3, pp. 10-157–10-160) NY: Matthew Bender and Co.

Roberts, J., and Hawk, B. (1980). *Legal rights primer for the handicapped: In and out of the classroom.* Novato, CA: Academic Therapy Publications.

Schifani, J. W., Anderson, R. M., and Odle, S. J. (1983). *Implementing learning in the least restrictive environment.* Baltimore: University Park Press.

Shrybman, J. A. (1982). *Due process in special education.* Rockville, MD: Aspen Systems Corporation.

Turnbull, A. P., and Schulz, J. B. (1979). *Mainstreaming handicapped students: A guide for the classroom teacher.* Boston: Allyn and Bacon.

Wallace, J. (Ed.). (1980). *Clarification of PL 94-142 for the administrator.* Philadelphia: Research for Better Schools.

Chapter 2

The Individualized Education Program and Related Services

Linda F. Bluth

One of the most widely discussed and most written about aspects of Public Law 94-142 is the Individualized Education Program (IEP). The IEP concept is not new, in that programs for handicapped children have often been based upon the premise that each handicapped child requires an individually tailored program in order to benefit from special education. The Education for All Handicapped Children Act of 1975 (Public Law 94-142), however, mandated that each handicapped child have this "individualized education program" (Education of the Handicapped Regulations, 1985).

For most new special education teachers and related service providers, the writing of IEPs is a task for which they have been inadequately prepared. Teachers who have provided children with exemplary individual programs often report that they were not trained in writing IEPs (Shrybman, 1982). In addition, the IEP is generally not a part of the training of related service providers, who are typically trained as clinicians and not specifically to work in an education system.

Related service providers often find difficulty using an IEP format. For example, "present level of performance" is often difficult to determine in the areas of medical services, parent counseling, school health services, and transportation, because in these areas there are no standardized measurement instruments for evaluating current functional levels.

Related services, in connection with an IEP, are services required to assist a handicapped child to benefit from special education (Education of the Handicapped Regulations, 1985). If a child does not need special education, he or she is not eligible for related services under Public Law 94-142.

For example, the child who is in the third grade and breaks a leg is not eligible for physical therapy or transportation as defined under PL 94-142.

Public Law 94-142 states that each public agency is responsible for initiating and conducting meetings for the purpose of developing, reviewing, and revising a handicapped child's individualized education program (Education of the Handicapped Regulations, 1985). It is important that an IEP development meeting be attended by all persons who have responsibility for the child's educational program. Because full attendance is not always feasible, it is essential that related service providers prepare a draft of their respective sections of the IEP after all the assessments have been conducted and that they be accountable for the implementation of their sections. The participants required to attend an IEP meeting are defined in federal regulations as follows:

1. A representative of the public agency, other than the child's teacher, who is qualified to provide, or supervise the provision of, special education.
2. The child's teacher.
3. One or both of the child's parents.
4. The child, when appropriate.
5. Other individuals at the discretion of the parent or agency.
6. Evaluation personnel.

For a handicapped child who is being evaluated for the first time, the public agency is required to ensure that a member of the evaluation team participate in the meeting *or* that the representative of the public agency, the child's teacher, or some other person who is knowledgeable about the evaluation procedures used with the child and familiar with the results of the evaluation is present at the meeting.

For the most productive meetings, it is essential that a multidisciplinary group of minimum size be present to focus on the development of the IEP based upon the strengths and weaknesses of the child. Assessment scores, observation reports, and anecdotal material are all important for this purpose.

The quality of parental involvement is essential in proceeding step by step through the IEP process. Federal law requires that "each public agency shall take steps to ensure that one or both of the parents of the handicapped child are present at each meeting or are afforded the opportunity to participate" (Education of the Handicapped Regulations, 1985).

CONTENTS OF AN IEP

The individualized education program for each child must include the following:

1. *A statement of the child's current levels of educational performance.* Information is obtained from the results of the evaluation process.

2. *A statement of annual goals, including short-term instructional objectives.* Annual goals include information based upon what it is the child will be able to do in light of the present levels of educational performance. The short-term objectives are those measurable statements that indicate steps needed to meet the annual goals.

3. *A statement of the specific special education and related services to be provided to the child, and the extent to which the child will be able to participate in regular education programs.* This issue is most often handled by recording the specific number of hours that a child will spend in special education and related services versus the number of hours in regular education. Time is most frequently recorded on a weekly or class period basis.

4. *The projected dates for initiation of services and the anticipated duration of the services.* The dates indicate when the specific services are to begin and when they will end. These dates are only projected, and changes can be made by conducting a review IEP meeting.

5. *Appropriate objective criteria and evaluation procedures and schedules for determining, on at least an annual basis, whether the short-term instructional objectives are being achieved.* This information is important in evaluating the benefit of specific services to the total education plan and is recorded and reviewed at least yearly.

STEPS IN THE IEP PROCESS

It is essential that related service providers be trained and knowledgeable about the steps required for completing the IEP process. These steps are discussed individually.

Identification

The identification of a child suspected of being handicapped is the first step in the process of delivery of service. Identification must be carefully considered, because it starts the process in motion. When a child is suspected of being handicapped, that child is screened and an evaluation may be initiated.

Evaluation

The purpose of evaluation is to determine whether or not the child is handicapped. This is the step that determines whether a child is eligible to receive special education and related services. Parental consent is required prior to assessment. All areas related to the suspected handicapping condition must be assessed by qualified examiners. A qualified examiner and a related service provider may or may not be the same person. The assessment results are important because they establish the need for service and answer questions related to eligibility for special education and related services.

After all evaluations are completed and it is determined that a child is handicapped, the next procedure is to determine the special education and related services needed. We must stress here that one of the most important procedural safeguards against evaluation bias is that "no single procedure is used as the sole criterion for determining an appropriate educational program for a child" (Education of the Handicapped Regulations, 1985). In addition, a multidisciplinary team conducts the appropriate assessments. This team includes at least one teacher or other specialist with knowledge in the area of suspected disability. When evaluations are completed and reviewed, the development of the IEP is initiated.

IEP Development

This is a comprehensive task requiring cooperation and sensitivity from the agency, parents, and all participants working on the development of the IEP. It is important to develop an IEP with consideration for direct and indirect services, length of service delivery, and setting for service delivery with emphasis placed on remediation of deficits. One should remember that the IEP does not always cover the child's entire educational program but is more like a prescriptive plan based upon assessment results. Each of the service providers should be comfortable with his or her section of the IEP.

The law requires that the IEP must be in place prior to service delivery, including parental approval. The IEP is important to all involved and most specifically the handicapped child, because it (1) indicates individual programming needs based on the unique needs of the child; (2) contains a record of all the services, their frequency, the service providers, and the service environment; (3) is a commitment for delivery of service; (4) provides for a measurement of accountability of all service providers; (5) provides for parental involvement; and (6) ensures continuity of programming.

The IEP meeting serves as a means of facilitating communication among the appropriate agency representatives and the parents. It enables all interested parties to develop and review annually the individualized requirements of a child's program and to work cooperatively to resolve areas of concern. The IEP document is a written record of all the services necessary to enable a handicapped child to receive special education and related services and can be appropriately considered a management tool. In addition to the functions mentioned, it serves as a compliance and monitoring instrument. If agreement about the IEP contents cannot be reached, the agency should inform the parents that they may seek to resolve their differences through a due process hearing.

Sometimes an agency and parents agree upon the basic IEP services but disagree about a section of the IEP, such as a particular related service. It is best in such instances to implement the agreed-upon sections of the IEP if both parties are in agreement and to work out that section of the IEP in question after the rest of the IEP has been approved.

Implementation

Implementation is the actual delivery of services (IEP contents) by all the required parties. This step requires coordination of all parties. Case management must be a part of the process, in order to coordinate all the components in a meaningful manner.

CONCLUSION

Related services are an important aspect of special education programming. For many students, related services maximize the opportunity to benefit from special education and attain a maximum level of independence. These services are best provided when they are recorded appropriately in the IEP form so that all parties are knowledgeable about the child's total individualized education program.

REFERENCES

Education of the Handicapped Regulations. (1985). 34 Code of Federal Regulations Part 300, Supplement 138.

Shrybman, J. A. (1982). *Due process in special education.* Rockville, MD: Aspen Systems Corporation.

PART II
RELATED SERVICES

Chapter 3

Audiology

Brad Friedrich

Historically, audiology programs have emphasized a number of service components in meeting the needs of hearing-impaired children. These components are incorporated into the definition of audiology in Public Law 94-142.

DEFINITION OF AUDIOLOGY SERVICES

The definition of audiology services in PL 94-142 is as follows:

1. The identification of children with hearing loss;
2. Determination of the range, nature, and degree of hearing loss, including referral for medical or other professional attention for the habilitation of hearing;
3. Provision of habilitative activities, such as language habilitation, auditory training, speech reading (lip reading), hearing evaluation, and speech conservation;
4. Creation and administration of programs for prevention of hearing loss;
5. Counseling and guidance of pupils, parents, and teachers regarding hearing loss; and
6. Determination of the child's need for group and individual amplification, selecting and fitting an appropriate aid, and evaluating the effectiveness of amplification. (Education of the Handicapped Regulations, 1985).

More recently, the audiologist has been involved increasingly in the direct delivery of habilitative and treatment services designed to optimize a child's use of residual hearing. As seen in the preceding definition, these services include auditory training, speech reading, speech conservation, and language development. They are also defined by Public Law 94-142 as being within the scope of audiology services.

RELATIONSHIP TO SPECIAL EDUCATION

Although the involvement of audiology in the educational process has changed in recent years, educational systems typically have not focused major attention on the provision of audiology services. Audiologists have assumed a more active role in the educational management of hearing-impaired children as members of multidisciplinary teams. Yet, in many instances the audiologist has served in no more than an adjunct role in the development and implementation of intervention strategies, both at the point of entry of the child to the educational environment and in the provision of ongoing services (Kenworthy, 1982). This fact is somewhat surprising in light of the prevalence of hearing impairment in the preschool and school-age population and the audiologist's role as the principle professional responsible for the evaluation of auditory function. Two factors appear to be chiefly responsible for the limited role of the school audiologist. First, a number of difficulties have been associated with the assessment of hearing impairment in young children, particularly in the presence of co-existing handicapping conditions. Nonetheless, audiological test techniques currently exist that permit the auditory status of the large majority of children to be determined regardless of age or handicapping condition (Friedrich, 1985). Second, the audiologist has functioned traditionally in the medical environment. Indeed, most audiologists continue to deliver services in health care settings today.

The mandates of federal and state legislative bodies have been largely responsible for increasing and improving the attention paid by audiologists to the education and habilitation of hearing-impaired children. Public Law 94-142, for example, has resulted in employment of audiologists by educational systems in significantly greater numbers. However, the actual number of audiologists in such settings is reported to be less than anticipated (American Speech-Language-Hearing Association, 1979; Garstecki, 1978; Ross, 1979). In addition, as Garstecki (1978) and Kenworthy (1982) point out, the role of the audiologist often remains limited. This problem reflects, at least in part, the various service models that educational systems have adopted for the provision of audiology services.

Nonetheless, the importance of audiology to the educational performance of hearing impaired children cannot be underestimated. Clinical audiological data are integral to educational, communicative, and vocational planning. Direct and strong relationships have been demonstrated to exist between the clinical data acquired in the audiologist's controlled test environment and the actual performance of children both communicatively and educationally. Of course, additional factors related to developmental status, behavior, and learning environment interact with the sensory deficit to determine ultimate achievement. Therefore, the audiologist must be prepared to be involved directly in assessment of performance outside the clinical environment as well.

The role of audiology in the educational management of children whose sole handicapping condition is hearing impairment is obvious. In such instances, the audiologist is likely to relate most frequently and directly to educators of the hearing impaired and to speech-language pathologists. The role of audiology is no less central, however, in the management of children who exhibit other handicapping conditions as well. The primary goal of the audiological evaluation is to determine the adequacy of a child's hearing for the development of linguistic and communicative skills that will permit academic progress (Friedrich, 1985). Yet, for a child with other handicaps, the audiologist must assist the various other professionals in understanding the child's hearing impairment in the context of his or her functioning in all spheres of development. The audiologist must join other multidisciplinary team members in ascertaining the relative impact of a child's disabilities on development and educational achievement.

The definition of audiology services in Public Law 94-142 also includes the creation and administration of programs for prevention of hearing impairment. Although audiologists in school settings are concerned primarily with children who exhibit communicatively handicapping impairments, they are also frequently responsible for screening programs and for assuring that diagnostic audiological evaluations are conducted to rule out hearing impairment in normally hearing children who may exhibit delays in speech and language development due to other factors, including cognitive deficits.

ELIGIBILITY FOR PROVISION OF RELATED SERVICES

Qualified audiologists typically are identified by one or more of the following professional credentials:

The *Certificate of Clinical Competence in Audiology (CCC-A)* is awarded by the American Speech-Language-Hearing Association, the scientific and professional organization representing audiologists and speech-language pathologists. The requirements for the CCC-A include completion of prescribed academic coursework (typically leading to a master's degree), clinical practicum clock hours, passing a national examination, and a supervised clinical fellowship year. The CCC-A is the most widely held and recognized credential for audiologists. It is required in the large majority of employment settings in which audiologists are found.

State licensure of audiologists currently exists in 36 states. State licensure requirements vary, although they frequently parallel those for the CCC-A. However, in all but five states with licensing laws, audiologists employed in public educational systems are exempt from licensure (American Speech-Language-Hearing Association, 1985).

State educational certification standards have been implemented at this time in only 21 states for personnel providing audiological services in public educational settings (American Speech-Language-Hearing Association,

1985). These certification standards usually are developed and administered by state departments of education. In many instances, they are less stringent than requirements for either the CCC-A or licensure. For example, a bachelor's degree rather than a master's degree is the minimal academic requirement in eight of the 21 states with audiologist certification requirements. Thus, disparities exist in many localities between the credentials required of audiologists in health care and education environments.

The American Speech-Language-Hearing Association also sponsors a voluntary accreditation program for clinical service programs in audiology and speech-language pathology. The program is administered by the Association's Professional Services Board (PSB). A number of educational systems in the nation have opted to seek accreditation of their audiological services.

OPTIONS IN SERVICE DELIVERY MODELS

The specific model of service delivery in audiology adopted by an educational system is determined primarily by whether the system chooses to provide diagnostic services in audiology. The comprehensive evaluation of auditory status depends, of course, upon the availability of a sound-treated test environment and an array of audiological equipment for the measurement of hearing and the analysis of hearing aids and other amplification devices. Many educational systems have found the capital expenditures associated with the provision of these services to be too great. As a consequence, three basic models of service delivery have evolved, although the scope of services rendered within individual programs varies widely.

First Model: No School-Provided Services

In the first model, no audiology services are offered by the educational system. Children often are seen for these services in a variety of clinical environments outside the school setting, such as hospitals, university clinics, private practices, and community agencies. In such instances, school personnel must establish contacts with audiological centers responsible for evaluation services and then must rely upon them to obtain and interpret vital clinical data. Many of these services are covered by family personal insurance plans or public assistance programs. In other instances, schools will purchase the services directly from audiological centers.

Under this model, specific intervention services such as auditory training, speech reading, and language development are delivered by other professional personnel in the school setting, including speech-language pathologists and educators. The American Speech-Language-Hearing Association (1984) has developed guidelines that identify competencies for the provision of aural rehabilitative services. Those guidelines recognize that overlap exists between professions and that similar services may be offered by more than one professional. Thus, this model of service delivery often denies school personnel the benefits of on-site audiological input into the educational management of hearing-impaired children on a continuous basis.

Second Model: School-Employed Audiologists

Other educational systems have chosen the second basic model for service delivery. They do not offer a diagnostic facility for audiology but do employ audiologists. The audiologists are responsible for the management of several aspects of a hearing-impaired child's educational program, which may include one or more of the following:

1. Development and implementation of programs for daily monitoring of hearing aid use and care.
2. Selection, adjustment, and evaluation of personal and group amplification systems (for example, FM transmission systems).
3. Provision of direct habilitative services, including auditory training, speech reading, speech conservation, and language development.
4. Provision of indirect consultative services to other school personnel (including teachers and speech-language pathologists) regarding appropriate modes of interaction and intervention with hearing-impaired children.
5. Staff development and in-service training.
6. Serving as a liaison with audiological centers responsible for the students outside the educational environment.

Third Model: School-Provided Diagnostic Services

Educational systems that choose to provide diagnostic services exemplify the third model. Commonly, a central diagnostic center is maintained for the entire system. Audiology services often are limited and are not as comprehensive, owing to financial and technical resource factors, as those available in health care and other settings; for example, auditory brainstem response testing, a well-established procedure that often requires sedation to assess infants and difficult-to-test children, is usually administered only in clinical settings with appropriate medical and technical resources. Nonetheless, service capabilities in educational diagnostic centers are often sufficient to permit at least the basic assessment of auditory function in all but the most difficult-to-test cases.

Frequently, children are followed by an audiologist in the community as well. At the request of parents, primary responsibility for on-going audiological management, including hearing aid selection, often rests with the clinical audiologist. This can lead to conflicts between the clinical audiologist and school personnel as to the interpretation of data as well as differences in the formulation of management plans and recommendations for individual children. In order to work satisfactorily, this model requires a high degree of cooperation between personnel in the educational and clinical environments.

IMPLICATIONS FOR IEP DEVELOPMENT

Upon determination that a child possesses a hearing impairment requiring special educational services, the individualized educational program (IEP) becomes the mechanism for defining those services, including audiology services. The IEP should specify goals and activities that are appropriate to support a particular child's educational program. The scope and frequency of the services will vary, depending upon the type and degree of the hearing impairment and the impact it has on the child's ability to function successfully in the classroom. The school audiologist should be assigned primary responsibility for the development of goals for his or her direct involvement with the child. In addition, the audiologist should be involved in the designation of appropriate objectives and frequency of service for other aspects of the educational program as written into the IEP, to ensure that they are appropriate to the child's hearing impairment. The audiologist may have more responsibility for the design of a program than for its direct implementation. Other professionals may be responsible for the delivery of the specific habilitative services.

An individualized education program for a hearing-impaired child should delineate clearly plans and goals related to the following audiology services:

1. A program of amplification monitoring. The plan should include daily troubleshooting, listening checks, and visual inspections to ensure that personal hearing aids and group amplification systems (such as FM transmission auditory training units) are in proper working order; periodic care of hearing aid(s) (for example, earmold cleaning and verification that instrument adjustments are correct and in accordance with audiological recommendations); and training of children to monitor and care for amplification devices themselves.

2. A plan for use of amplification in the educational setting. This plan should include designation of time periods for use of both personal and group systems, particularly when their use may be limited by a child's level of cognitive functioning or by involvement in other activities that preclude or interfere with hearing aid use (such as physical therapy). Specific classroom activities should be identified for which auditory training units may be more crucial, in order to ensure optimal auditory input to the child. The use of FM systems with the direct audio input option of personal hearing aids should be clearly stated in the IEP.

3. A program for facilitating a child's adjustment, including initial acceptance, to amplification. Utilization of behavioral modification techniques
should be incorporated as appropriate.

4. Assignment of preferential seating in group learning and listening situations in accordance with a child's hearing impairment to ensure optimal
access to both auditory and visual cues for communication.

5. Modification of the acoustic environment to reduce ambient noise,
extraneous noises, and detrimental effects of reverberation that may
interfere with a hearing-impaired child's reception of spoken messages.

6. Specific intervention services delivered directly by the audiologist,
including auditory training, speech reading instruction, speech conservation, speech production training, and language development. Treatment
goals and frequency of service should be clearly designated.

7. Designation of any required audiological services that are to be procured
outside the educational environment.

ISSUES, CONCERNS, AND RECOMMENDATIONS

A number of issues and concerns surround the provision of audiology services in education. First, despite the impetus provided by legal mandates and
the advances of recent years, audiology as a related service is characterized
by considerable inconsistency among educational systems. This inconsistency reflects the myriad of service models and options and the variability
in professional qualifications required to provide services. Kenworthy (1982)
has concluded that audiology still is not an integral part of the educational
process. Only a few systems offer truly comprehensive services for both the
evaluation and management of hearing-impaired children. Thus, the specific
manner in which audiology relates to special education is still emerging at
this time.

Second, both Friedrich (1985) and Kenworthy (1982) have suggested
that hearing impairment frequently assumes a position of secondary importance in the educational management of children, particularly in the presence of cognitive and physical disabilities. In instances, the identification of
children with communicatively and educationally handicapping hearing
impairments has been unnecessarily compromised with concomitant delays
in educational placement and the provision of inappropriate services. This
problem remains a central concern for those individuals providing audiology services. The magnitude of the problem is increased when one considers current demographic data that suggest that more than 30 per cent of
hearing-impaired children studied in the Annual Survey of Hearing-
Impaired Children (conducted by Gallaudet College) exhibit one or more
additional handicapping conditions (Karchmer, 1985). Karchmer carefully
points out that the survey probably underestimates the actual number of

multiply-handicapped hearing-impaired children who require specialized educational services.

Third, as alluded to previously, the provision of audiology services in the educational environment is necessarily influenced by the fact that the services are both educational and medical in nature. Audiology services, particularly those related to diagnosis and evaluation, will probably remain largely in the clinical environment. Clinical facilities are likely to continue to be the only ones with the fiscal and technical resources sufficient to provide comprehensive diagnostic services, particularly in view of the important role of medicine in diagnosis and management of hearing impairment. Indeed, most hearing-impaired children are identified outside the educational environment and, in many instances, prior to entry into any educational program. The field of audiology must be prepared to bridge the gap between the two settings and fully to recognize hearing impairment as both a health problem and a communicative and academic problem.

In light of cost factors associated with diagnostic services and the general availability of those services in clinical facilities in most areas, educational administrators might most wisely opt for the adoption of service delivery models that emphasize the educational process and the direct impact audiology may have on the learning of hearing-impaired children. Kenworthy (1982) suggests, for example, that audiology has an expanded role to serve in monitoring the use of amplification devices in the classroom. Garstecki (1978) reports that few audiologists working in school settings provide amplification monitoring on a consistent basis. A number of investigators have documented the high number (estimates range as high as 40 to 60 per cent) of malfunctioning personal hearing aids and group amplification systems in schools on a daily basis (Coleman, 1972; Gaeth and Lounsbury, 1966; Hoversten, 1981; Kemker, McConnell, Logan, and Green, 1979; Northern, McChord, Fischer, and Evans, 1972; Sinclair and Freeman, 1981).

Similarly, efforts should be undertaken to optimize use of residual hearing through better design and control of the acoustic environment in classrooms. Many classrooms have high noise levels and poor reverberation characteristics (Olsen, 1981), but few school systems have chosen to examine and systematically modify problem listening environments.

Expanded in-service training and professional staff development by audiologists is also crucial. Kenworthy (1982) reports that a majority of regular education personnel encounter hearing-impaired children in the classroom. A large majority of those teachers report that they have insufficient information regarding hearing impairment and amplification.

Finally, a clear definition of the roles and responsibilities of the audiologist in the educational and clinical environments is necessary to minimize potential conflicts and the confusion that may otherwise result for teachers, professionals, and families. Role definition should help foster positive and constructive professional relationships and contribute to greater consistency among educational systems in the provision of audiology services. Although consistency is a desirable outcome, specific models for service delivery have to respond to specific situations as well.

REFERENCES

American Speech-Language-Hearing Association. (1979). Survey of audiological service and certification patterns in the schools. Washington, D.C.: ASHA.

American Speech-Language-Hearing Association. (1984). Definition of and competencies for aural rehabilitation. *ASHA, 26*, 37–41.

American Speech-Language-Hearing Association. (1985). State education consultant survey. Washington, D.C.: ASHA.

Coleman, R. (1972). Stability of children's hearing aids in an acoustic preschool. Final report. Project 522466, Grant No. OEG-4-71-0060. Washington, D.C.: U.S. Department of Health, Education and Welfare.

Education of the Handicapped Regulations. (1985). 34 Code of Federal Regulations Part 300, Supplement 138.

Friedrich, B. (1985). The state of the art in audiologic evaluation and management. In E. Cherow (Ed.), *Hearing-impaired children and youth with developmental disabilities.* Washington, D.C.: Gallaudet College Press.

Gaeth, J., & Lounsbury, E. (1966). Hearing aids and children in elementary schools. *Journal of Speech and Hearing Disorders, 31*, 283–289.

Garstecki, D. (1978). Survey of school audiologists. *ASHA, 20*, 291–296.

Hoversten, G. (1981). A public school audiology program: amplification maintenance, auditory management, and in-service education. In F. Bess, B. Freeman, & J. Sinclair (Eds.), *Amplification in education.* Washington, D.C.: Alexander Graham Bell Association.

Karchmer, M. (1985). A demographic perspective. In E. Cherow (Ed.), *Hearing-impaired children and youth with developmental disabilities.* Washington, D.C.: Gallaudet College Press.

Kemker, F., McConnell, F., Logan, S., & Green, B. (1979). A field study of children's hearing aids in a school environment. *Language, Speech and Hearing Services in the Schools, 10*, 47–53.

Kenworthy, O. (1982). Integration of assessment and management processes: Audiology as an educational program. In B. Campbell & V. Baldwin (Eds.), *Severely handicapped hearing impaired students: Strengthening service delivery.* Baltimore: Paul H. Brookes Publishing Co.

Northern, J., McChord, W., Fischer, E., & Evans, P. (1972). Hearing services in residential schools for the deaf. *Maico Audiological Library Series, 11*, 16–18.

Olsen, W. (1981). The effects of noise and reverberation on speech intelligibility. In F. Bess, B. Freeman, & J. Sinclair (Eds.), *Amplification in education.* Washington, D.C.: Alexander Graham Bell Association.

Ross, M. (1979). The audiologist in the schools. *ASHA, 21*, 858–862.

Sinclair, J., & Freeman, B. (1981). The status of classroom amplification in American education. In F. Bess, B. Freeman, & J. Sinclair (Eds.), *Amplification in education.* Washington, D.C.: Alexander Graham Bell Association.

Chapter 4

Counseling Services

Janie R. Friedlander

Counseling services have traditionally been an integral part of school organization. The school counselor works with children on self-understanding, career development, and career education. In many schools, the counseling function of school psychologists may well be performed by school counselors (Reynolds and Birch, 1977).

Counselors also assist children with educational and social adjustment. In addition, they collaborate with teachers in developing behavior management plans for children. Turnbull and Schulz (1979) observe that counselors have various roles to play in the implementation of mainstreaming.

DEFINITION OF COUNSELING SERVICES

Counseling services are defined in Public Law 94-142 as "services provided by qualified social workers, psychologists, guidance counselors, or other qualified personnel." The intent of providing counseling, as with any related service, is to assist a handicapped child to benefit from special education. The ultimate goal of counseling within a school setting should, therefore, be generally to improve a child's behavioral adjustment and control skills in order to make the child more available for participation in the educational program.

RELATIONSHIP TO SPECIAL EDUCATION

Counseling services are to be provided when an educationally handicapped child requires this support in order to benefit from the assigned special education instruction program. Counseling can, therefore, be recommended in the following situations:

1. When a child receives his or her primary education in a regular education classroom, and leaves that classroom for a period during the day in order to receive some form of special education instruction (such as speech and language therapy). Although the primary disability is not necessarily one relating to social or emotional disturbance, the child requires counseling services in order to develop social or behavioral skills necessary to benefit from special education.

2. When a child receives his or her primary education in a self-contained special education class, not specifically for emotional or social needs, and requires counseling services to benefit from special education.

3. When a child's primary education is provided in a special education setting where the curriculum is specifically designed for children displaying symptoms of emotional disturbance and the child requires counseling services to benefit from special education.

ELIGIBILITY FOR RELATED SERVICE PROVISION

Because the term counseling can be subject to many interpretations, it seems essential that each state education agency (SEA) and each local education agency (LEA) develop specific, written criteria to be met before this related service can be recommended. The decision to provide counseling as a related service must be made at an individualized education program (IEP) meeting. It is essential to obtain input from qualified personnel in order to determine the necessity as well as the extent of the service. Qualified professionals may include the school psychologist, psychiatrist, social worker, and guidance counselor. Input can also be provided by other professionals who have contact with the child, such as the teacher, the pediatrician, and a private clinician. The decision to recommend counseling should be based on written diagnostic reports that document the child's current social and emotional status. Documentation can include written observation over time as well as formal projective testing techniques.

Although it is not a requirement that a child's primary disability be a serious emotional disturbance in order to qualify for counseling service, it would seem helpful to use the definition of "seriously emotionally disturbed" to determine the need for counseling at the school level.

According to Public Law 94-142, "seriously emotionally disturbed" is explained as follows:

(i) The term means a condition exhibiting one or more of the following characteristics over a long period and to a marked degree, which adversely affects educational performance.
   (a) An inability to learn which cannot be explained by intellectual, sensory or health factors;
   (b) An inability to build or maintain satisfactory interpersonal relationships with peers and teachers;
   (c) Inappropriate types of behaviors or feelings under normal circumstances;
   (d) A general pervasive mood of unhappiness or depression; or
   (e) A tendency to develop physical symptoms or fears associated with personal or school problems.
(ii) The term applies to children who are schizophrenic. The term does not apply to children who are socially maladjusted, unless it is determined that they are seriously emotionally disturbed. (Education of the Handicapped Regulations, 1985).

COUNSELING VERSUS PSYCHOTHERAPY

One of the related services included in the regulations of Public Law 94-142 is medical services for diagnostic or evaluative purposes (Education of the Handicapped Regulations, 1985).

It is the restriction that medical services be only for diagnosis and evaluative purposes that has raised much confusion and debate for state and local school systems. Counseling services are defined in the law by the profession of the service provider (psychologist, social worker, or school counselor). Psychotherapy has been considered by many SEAs to be a medical service and therefore not recommended or paid for by a school system.

Court decisions in Connecticut and Montana have recently recognized psychotherapy as a related, not medical service and have ordered LEAs to provide this service without cost to the child or parent (Handicapped Students and Special Education, 1984). Relative to educational programming, these court decisions did not specifically identify the personnel to provide psychotherapy as a related service and apparently have left this decision to the LEAs. It seems imperative, therefore, for each SEA and LEA to develop specific written criteria regarding recommendation of this service and also to define the staff who will act as service providers.

Social workers as well as psychologists who work in school systems are often trained in counseling techniques. Psychotherapy, defined as a "psychological service" or "counseling service," may therefore be provided during the school day, by school personnel, as well as by private psychiatrists and clinical psychologists.

OPTIONS IN SERVICE DELIVERY MODELS

Several techniques for providing counseling in the school setting can be considered. The type of direct or indirect service chosen is to be based on the specific needs of the individual child. Following are brief descriptions of each.

Consultation

Consultation services can be provided to the classroom teacher by the school psychologist, social worker, or counselor. This is not a direct service to the child. The professional providing the service may supply input regarding an individual child or may offer suggestions to the teacher about classroom management techniques.

Classroom Meetings

Classroom meetings involve an entire class during a specified period of the school day. The service provider and the teacher co-lead the meeting, encouraging the children to participate. The goal of a class meeting is to develop better communication, behavioral adjustment, and control skills as well as to improve interpersonal relationship skills.

Small Group Counseling

Small group counseling sessions can be conducted with the children. The size of the group should be determined on the basis of age as well as the severity of the disability. Specific topics can be the focus of the meetings. These topics may include peer interaction, verbalization of feelings as they relate to the school experience, test taking strategies, and feelings about being handicapped. The group should be led by a school social worker, psychologist, or counselor.

Individual Counseling

Individual counseling sessions can be scheduled between a child and an appropriate staff person, such as a social worker, school psychologist, or counselor. The staff member responsible for delivery of the service should possess expertise directly related to the IEP objectives as well as to the severity of the problem. Individual counseling should be considered a vehicle to be used to help the child benefit from his or her special education program.

Parent Training

Training can be offered to the parents of children enrolled in self-contained classes for the emotionally disturbed or of infants and toddlers receiving special education instruction services. Possible topics include extension of services and techniques into the home (for example, behavior management techniques) and specific topics suggested by the parents.

IMPLICATIONS FOR IEP DEVELOPMENT

When counseling is recommended as a related service, the service provider must be designated on the IEP. The degree of severity of behaviors exhibited by the child will primarily determine the degree of specialization required by the service provider. The most common service providers within the school system are social workers, psychologists, and guidance counselors. These service providers possess various skills.

A school social worker is trained in group and individual counseling techniques, outside agency intervention, development of a social history for a child, and crisis intervention.

A guidance counselor is trained in career guidance, parent intervention, group process, and the teaching of test taking skills.

A school psychologist is trained in delivering psychodiagnostic evaluative techniques, group and individual counseling, crisis intervention, and outside agency intervention.

When the IEP committee determines the need for counseling as a related service, long-range goals and specific short-term objectives must be part of the IEP. The service provider as well as the extent (time period) and duration of service are to be specified. Goals and objectives are to be directly derived from the IEP statements describing the child's current levels of social, emotional, and behavioral functioning as they relate to educational progress. The nature of the counseling service is to respond directly to the specific objectives stated in the IEP.

When the intervention technique is decided upon, the name of the service provider is to be specified and written in the appropriate section of the IEP. The choice of service provider should be based on the type of service being recommended as well as the expertise of the professional. When the nature of a child's problems has been identified, a determination should be made as to which qualified personnel should provide the counseling service.

Techniques for evaluating the child's progress and ultimate achievement of the goals and objectives and the estimated date for acquisition of the objective are to be determined by the IEP committee.

In summary, the following sequence should be used to develop an IEP for a child who requires counseling as a related service:

1. *Assess the present level of performance.* Descriptors are to be stated in behavioral terms. Specific descriptions of both strengths and weaknesses should be included. Examples: "child displays age-appropriate social

interaction skills"; "child displays physically aggressive behaviors toward peers"; "child does not establish eye contact."

2. *Develop the goals.* Long-term goals are to relate directly to the child's present level of performance. They are to be global in nature. Examples: "child will develop appropriate behavioral adjustment and control skills"; "child will develop age-appropriate social interaction skills."

3. *Develop the objectives.* Short-term objectives are to be written in behavioral terms. Examples: "child will remain seated for 5 consecutive minutes"; "child will play appropriately with peers for 8 to 10 minutes"; "child will eliminate head banging behavior."

4. *Select the service provider and specify extent of service.* Identify the provider at the time of IEP development. Specific consideration should be given to the individual expertise of the various staff members trained to provide the counseling service. In addition, it should be noted that the child with more severe behaviors will probably need more frequent services.

5. *Establish the criteria for evaluation.* The measure for determining the achievement of each objective is to be specified. It should be a specific measure of the reduction of inappropriate behavior or the development of a more socially appropriate behavior. An example is a frequency chart indicating a 25 per cent decrease in head banging behavior.

Table 4–1 contains examples of information that might be supplied in an IEP for a child who requires counseling services.

ISSUES, CONCERNS, AND RECOMMENDATIONS

The definition of counseling as a related service in the school setting raises several issues. It seems crucial for state education agencies to develop strict definitions and guidelines for the local education agencies, because children are referred to school professionals for this service.

One major concern involves defining counseling in educational terms. Frequently, counseling is equated with psychotherapy, but in a school setting these two processes must be separated. Psychotherapy often implies a long-term commitment, and its ultimate goals may be varied. When counseling is recommended in an IEP, the goals and objectives are specifically related to improving academic performance, since the behaviors to be modified in the counseling situation must have an adverse effect on educational achievement. Treatment is then recommended to alleviate difficulties in the school setting. It seems most important for SEAs, LEAs, and individual professionals to be made aware of the difference between these two concepts. In-service staff training would probably be an effective means of educating school personnel about this issue.

Table 4–1.   Sample IEP Information

1. **Current level of educational performance**	Short attention span Unable to participate in group activity Physically aggressive with peers
2. **Long-term goals**	The child will develop age-appropriate behavioral and adjustment and control skills The child will improve interpersonal relationship skills
3. **Short-term objectives**	The child will be able to attend to a task until completion The child will participate in a small group activity, demonstrating appropriate behaviors, e.g., taking turns, sharing The child will participate in a small group activity and demonstrate no physically aggressive behaviors toward group members
4. **Service provider/ extent of service**	The service provider will be the school social worker. The extent of service is one 40-minute period, once each week, in a group counseling session of 4 to 6 children for 6 months
5. **Evaluation criteria**	Teacher or school social worker observation reports Child checklist completed by the teacher or school social worker

Educational requirements for professionals are another issue that must be addressed. Traditionally, many student social workers receive training in the process of therapy/counseling, as do guidance counselors. Postgraduate programs therefore need to focus on counseling skills within a school system, as opposed to those needed in a more traditional psychotherapy situation.

Because most postgraduate school psychology programs have a major focus on evaluative and diagnostic procedures, and more school psychologists are called upon to provide counseling as a related service, it is imperative for universities to require counseling courses as part of the curriculum. Furthermore, an integral portion of each postgraduate student's internship should be a counseling experience. The student should be allowed to observe as well as take part in individual and group counseling situations in the school.

Another issue revolves around the assignment of counseling cases. There is a question as to whether one profession may be better equipped to deal with certain behaviors and symptoms. This question relates to the issue of training at the postgraduate level. Perhaps there should be some uniformity of skills taught for those counselors working in a school. This final concern overlaps the issue of determining which counseling situation a child requires (that is, individual, group, or class meeting). If a child's IEP states that small group counseling is recommended, but there are no existing group sessions in the school, how are the child's goals and objectives to be met? Should the child therefore receive individual therapy until an appropriate group can be formed?

These issues require specific answers. Although each case should be decided individually, a specific definition would result in less confusion and misinterpretation of the law. The formation of a specific, detailed policy in keeping with Public Law 94-142 and state regulations is recommended. SEAs and LEAs must work together to formulate these policies and procedures so that they can logically fit into a school environment while remaining in compliance with legal mandates.

REFERENCES

Education of the Handicapped Regulations. (1985). 34 Code of Federal Regulations Part 300, Supplement 138.

Handicapped Students and Special Education. (1984). Rosemount, MN: Data Research, Inc.

Reynolds, M. C., & Birch, J. W. (1977). Teaching exceptional children in all America's schools. Reston, VA: The Council for Exceptional Children.

Turnbull, A. P., & Schulz, J. B. (1979). Mainstreaming handicapped students: A guide for the classroom teacher. Boston: Allyn and Bacon, Inc.

Chapter 5

Early Identification

Maryanne Conlon Ralls

Awareness of the necessity of educating handicapped children as early as possible was affirmed by the United States Congress with the passage of the Education for All Handicapped Children Act of 1975, Public Law 94-142. In its investigations prior to passage of the Act, Congress found many surprising facts regarding the status of special education in the United States. In addition to the numbers of handicapped children being underserved or totally excluded from school, it was determined that a great number of children were failing in regular education programs because of undetected handicaps. As a result, the federal law included "the early identification and assessment of handicapping conditions in children" as one of its related services. Congress intended that these children with undetected handicaps be found, identified as handicapped, and placed in appropriate programs. In addition, handicapped children not already in school would also be found, assessed, and placed in programs appropriate to their needs.

DEFINITION OF EARLY IDENTIFICATION

According to the regulation implementing Public Law 94-142, early identification and assessment of disabilities in children is defined as "the implementation of a formal plan for identifying a disability as early as possible in a child's life" (Education of the Handicapped Regulations, 1985).

The intent of early identification is therefore to locate and identify handicapped children as soon as possible, as is clearly indicated in both the federal statute and the implementing regulations. As noted in the comments accompanying the regulations, simply locating and identifying these children is not enough. They must also be provided "services to minimize the effects of such conditions."

RELATIONSHIP TO SPECIAL EDUCATION

The relationship between special education and any of the related services is quite clear in the Public Law 94-142 regulations. "Related services" are support services provided to children in order that they may benefit from special education. Although the main focus of early identification is to locate and identify children and to place them in programs appropriate to their needs, it is not the only purpose. For children already in a special education program, early identification becomes the vehicle for identifying any secondary disabilities or needs and addressing them in already existing programs. Hence, early identification has a two-fold relationship to special education. Early identification is the avenue by which a child enters special education as well as the means to add or change services provided to children already in special education programs.

ELIGIBILITY FOR RELATED SERVICE PROVISION

The federal regulations explicitly state that in order to be classified as handicapped, a child must have one of the identified impairments and must be in need of special education. Also, in order to receive a related service, a child must need the service to support his special education program. Confusion obviously arises when the related service of early identification is in question. Early identification is generally regarded as a service performed to enable a child to enter special education programs.

OPTIONS IN SERVICE DELIVERY MODELS

Delivery of early identification services falls into three stages: location, identification, and placement.

Location

With the passage of Public Law 94-142, the location of handicapped children became of paramount concern. State and local education agencies set up Child Find offices to locate handicapped children not yet in school and children who may possibly be handicapped. Numerous Child Find offices began a media blitz, with television ads, radio ads, and billboards becoming commonplace. Perhaps the most effective method of locating handicapped children continues to be the education of the community. The staff in Child Find offices provides valuable information to the community. Through meetings and workshops, professionals in many fields related to education learn to identify potential problems and obtain assistance for the children in their care. Personnel in social services and juvenile services agencies as well as the medical profession are now becoming more aware of the signs and symptoms of potential handicapping conditions. Teachers and administrators are more aware of services available to children and know how to help parents obtain these services. Although the location of handicapped children continues to be important, it is only the first stage in early identification (Meyen, 1982).

Identification

Once a child with a suspected handicapping condition is located, he or she must move into the identification stage of early identification. This stage begins with the referral process, which is usually based on the suspicion of the presence of a handicapping condition. Referrals may come from a variety of sources, including parents, teachers, medical personnel, and community agencies. Referrals are often received in a central location by the personnel responsible for early identification services. The team involved in the process should be multidisciplinary and should be experienced in dealing with preschool children as well as in the identification of handicapping conditions and in preschool special education programming. Especially important to this team are the disciplines of special education, psychology, social work, and speech/language. Although all disciplines may not be necessary for every child, the input of each is valuable in overall programming.

Upon receipt of a referral to the early identification services team, a case manager can be assigned to begin the screening process. The case manager is responsible for making the decisions necessary to process the case. If the referral was not made by the parents, they must be contacted for their approval. Information must then be gathered relative to the areas of the suspected handicap. For screening of young children, information is needed in all areas of development: cognition, language, motor, self-help, and social-emotional. The case manager obtains available information in each area and prepares the case for presentation to the early identification team. The team then decides whether sufficient appropriate information for determination of a handicapping condition has been obtained or additional assessments are needed.

After the determination that additional assessments are necessary, early identification moves into the assessment phase. The team decides what assessments are necessary and who is responsible for each. The case manager is responsible for ensuring that all assessments are completed in a timely fashion. Formal and informal assessment information is needed to assist in the decision-making.

Placement

Upon completion of all of the requested assessments, early identification moves into the placement stage. The early identification team must review the assessments and determine whether the child has a handicapping condition. Next, the educational and related services needs of the child must be determined. Finally, an individualized education program (IEP) must be developed and a placement must be determined.

Placement options for young children take different forms. Programs may be home-based, center-based, or a combination of both (Jordan, Hayden, Karnes, and Wood, 1979). Home-based programs involve visits by an itinerant teacher to the home, several days per week, to work with the child and the parents. The itinerant teacher instructs the parents in methods for working with the child on maintaining mastered skills, and also provides direct instruction to the child. Center-based programs offer a variety of services. In addition to direct instruction, centers usually offer an array of related services. A child may attend the center for varying times, from an hour or more up to five full days per week, depending upon the severity of the handicapping condition.

IMPLICATIONS FOR IEP DEVELOPMENT

As with all handicapped children, placement in an early identification program is dependent upon the development of an individualized education program (IEP). The content of the IEP must address the deficits identified during the assessment phase. The decision to place the child in a home-based program or a center-based program depends upon the services needed as identified in the IEP. The placement of handicapped children through the early identification process must be in accordance with all federal and state regulations governing IEP development and placement. These regulations require a review of the IEP on at least an annual basis.

ISSUES, CONCERNS, AND RECOMMENDATIONS

Although public awareness of handicapped children has increased dramatically during the last decade, more attention is needed. Negative attitudes about the handicapped, especially young children, need to be changed so that early identification programs may be expanded and improved. Professional training should also be expanded so that educators may become better equipped to instruct young handicapped children (Fine and Swift, 1986).

To assist the psychologist and the special educator in the early identification process, more reliable standardized assessment instruments must be developed. Further research will also lead to the development of effective, expanded programming. The continuation of Child Find programs and early identification procedures will enable young handicapped children to benefit from educational services.

REFERENCES

Education of the Handicapped Regulations. (1985). 34 Code of Federal Regulations Part 300, Supplement 138.

Fine, M. & Swift, C. (1986). Young handicapped children: Their prevalence and experiences with early intervention services. *Early Childhood*, 10, 73–83.

Jordan, J., Hayden, A., Karnes, M., & Wood, M. (Eds.) (1979). *Early childhood education for exceptional children*. Virginia: Council for Exceptional Children.

Meyen, E. (1982). *Exceptional children in today's schools*. Colorado: Love Publishing Company.

Chapter **6**

Medical Services

Dennis Whitehouse

The term "medical services," as used in this chapter, refers to services provided by a licensed physician. Although other professionals, such as doctors of osteopathy and nurse practitioners, may provide similar services, the understood requirement is for a licensed medical practitioner to provide these services. In some situations, such as in the diagnosis of children with severe emotional handicaps, the requirement may include certification in a particular specialty, such as psychiatry.

DEFINITION OF MEDICAL SERVICES

Medical services, as defined in Public Law 94-142, are services provided by a licensed physician to determine a medically related handicapping condition that results in the affected child's need for special education and related services (Education of the Handicapped Regulations, 1985).

The first important qualification is that these medical services must be for diagnostic purposes only. They do not qualify as funded services if they are given for therapeutic reasons. An exception to this is that medical services are permitted for the habilitation of hearing, speech, and language problems, if needed. Although diagnostic procedures may lead to therapeutic recommendations, no recommendations can be made without prior diagnosis.

RELATIONSHIP TO SPECIAL EDUCATION

For the majority of handicapping conditions defined by Public Law 94-142, there is a difference in function between a handicapped and a non-handicapped child. In some cases this difference may be the result of a prior disease that has led to changes in the physiological state of the brain. More often these conditions exemplify variations in brain function that are inherited and result in a neurologically determined difference in function, whether motor, sensory, cognitive, or behavioral. Although secondary environmental factors may modify these basic functions, there is nevertheless a neurological substrate that can be regarded as basically a medical problem. It follows that all qualified examiners engaged in the diagnosis of these handicapping conditions are also engaged in evaluating the complex multiple functions or dysfunctions of the motor, sensory, cognitive, or behavioral systems that compose each child's particular handicap. Each diagnostician will be overlapping the evaluations of his or her colleagues in all these dimensions, with each specialist contributing major diagnostic components in his or her own field and minor ones in other areas. It is this overlap in diagnostic criteria that provides the major value of the interdisciplinary approach, leading to a clearer diagnosis.

ELIGIBILITY FOR RELATED SERVICE PROVISION

The first requirement of a medical evaluation is to ascertain the precise reason for the child's referral. This inquiry is even more relevant when a physician is seeing a child for the purpose of assisting with educational procedures. Aside from the known fact that a potential handicapping condition exists and can be recognized as medically based, there has to be an added reason for the medical evaluation. One reason for asking for medical services can be uncertainty about diagnosis in areas outside the expertise of the other team members. The psychologist may, for example, ask for a neurological examination to establish accurate diagnosis in an area other than intelligence testing, such as motor, sensory or speech and hearing. This second opinion may be unnecessary if the areas in question fall within the expertise of another member of the educational team, such as the audiologist, speech pathologist, physical therapist, or occupational therapist.

A second reason for referral could be to establish a physical basis for the findings, namely that the handicapping condition is indeed a condition defined by Public Law 94-142 and not the result of cultural or environmental factors. In this respect the medical evaluation is more firmly organically based than many other evaluations, and the physician may be able to confirm the organic nature of the problem. Needless to say, establishment of organic nature is not necessarily the only purpose for these evaluations, because environmental factors must inevitably impinge on the handicapped child, just as primary or secondary emotional problems may be playing a part in addition to the handicapping condition. It is clearly important that the child's behavioral aspects should be evaluated, and the physician may have a valuable role, in conjunction with the other members of the team, in establishing the nature of such behavioral interference.

A third reason for referral of a child for medical evaluation is to diagnose or rule out other medical disorders that may interfere with learning. Although the primary handicapping conditions as defined by Public Law 94-142 mostly represent neurological disorders or dysfunctions, non-neurological conditions are also included, such as severe hearing and visual impairments and orthopedic problems. Chronic health conditions that adversely affect a child's educational performance are also listed in Public Law 94-142 under the category "other health impaired." This category includes children:

(i)   having an autistic condition which is manifested by severe communication and other developmental and educational problems; or
(ii) having limited strength, vitality or alertness, due to chronic or acute health problems such as a heart condition, tuberculosis, rheumatic fever, nephritis, asthma, sickle cell anemia, hemophilia, epilepsy, lead poisoning, leukemia, or diabetes, which adversely affects a child's educational performance. (Education of the Handicapped Regulations, 1985).

In these medical conditions, the physician may be the prime diagnostician on the team and an essential part of the evaluation.

Relationship to Parents

The relationship between the physician and parent when a child has been referred for medical services must come under the normal physician-patient guidelines. It is implicit in this evaluation that the client with whom the physician is dealing is the child and his or her parents or guardian, and not necessarily only the school. For emotional reasons, this physician-client relationship must be maintained and may even involve problems with confidentiality. The normal procedure is for the physician to meet for a final conference with parents and to review the diagnostic profile and recommendations with them. This final conference will also include the child, if he or she is old enough and can understand and benefit from the meeting. Most physicians working in this field, and most clinics, hold the professional conference first and the parent conference subsequently. The advantage of this order is that parents can then be given all the information, including recommendations that have been made at the professional conference and are likely to be implemented or considered for implementation. In the majority of cases, this procedure works very well with no complications. The final parent conference is then followed by sending a written report to those concerned. In some cases, parents do not accept this procedure and are anxious about disclosing information to the school. The physician must agree to keep certain information confidential and will have no problems in doing so if the information is not relevant to the case. When the confidential information is relevant, the situation is more difficult, and the only recommendation that can be made is that of pursuing a course of complete honesty in dealing with all concerned.

Because related services are mandated by Public Law 94-142 and implemented at the school level using public funds, all provisions of Public Law 94-142 apply and the parents as well as the school have certain rights. Referral from school personnel implies a requirement to provide a report and recommendations to them. A conference called for and held by the school, involving the physician, also mandates that parents should be invited. In all cases, whether the child is referred by the school system or privately, the physician should obtain permission from parents to carry out the procedures. Permission is needed for examination of the child, to talk with school personnel, and subsequently to send a report to the school.

Types of Medical Services

Traditionally the *psychiatrist* has been held responsible for the care of the mentally retarded. The origin of this practice may be due, in part, to early ideas of the separation of mind and body. Most mental retardation administrations have come under mental rather than physical health divisions. Mental retardation and autism originally were problems likely to be referred to the psychiatrist.

The first descriptions of learning disabilities came from *neurologists* in the mid and late 19th century from studies of adults who had suffered brain injury. Broca (1865) first described inability to speak as a result of brain injury to the left pre-motor area. Soon afterwards Wernicke (1874) described adults who had lost the ability to comprehend language and who had also suffered brain injury to the left side of the brain, particularly in the posterior temporal area. Berlin (1887) described six adults who had lost the ability to read following what was thought to be mild brain injury. Only in 1895 did Hinshelwood describe a child who was thought to have a congenital inability to read and who was recognized as not being retarded. Throughout this period there were many other reports of adults with different "learning disabilities" of neurological origin, leading to a very active continuing interest in these disabilities on the part of neurologists.

Since the development of pediatrics as a specialty, the *pediatrician* has been the physician who follows the growth and development of children and is, consequently, in a position to first recognize deviations in development. Pediatricians have continued to follow children through adolescence and into adult life and have been able to watch the evolution of handicapping conditions.

Generally, the psychiatrist may concentrate more on behavior and may not be as familiar with underlying learning processes. The neurologist may be more concerned with learning and not as concerned with underlying behavioral consequences. Unfortunately, the pediatrician may not be well trained in developmental medicine and may not have adequate neurological or psychiatric background to be familiar with these complex problems.

It readily becomes clear that no one professional discipline can claim to be the primary provider of diagnostic medical services. In most cases the physician, whether psychiatrist, neurologist, or pediatrician, will be asked to carry out the diagnostic procedures mandated. This means that facilities for the provision of these medical services will vary from state to state and city to city. In most cases, a number of recognized physicians known to work in this area will be willing to function as members of an interdisciplinary team for evaluating suspected handicapping conditions.

OPTIONS IN SERVICE DELIVERY MODELS

Medical services can be provided at a number of different sites. An appropriate specialist might provide diagnostic services in his or her office. A physician may provide this service in a special outpatient clinic at a local hospital. A third site might be in a teaching hospital as part of a university program. These services can be provided in a department of psychiatry, neurology, or pediatrics. In some states, specific clinics are set up for diagnostic purposes, either in a private facility such as a university or private hospital or in a public health facility. These clinics may go under many different titles, all pertaining to the diagnosis and evaluation of children. The clinics usually consist of a medically oriented team but may also include many professionals in addition to the physician. In the past, most of these teams were led by a physician director, although the trend today is for other professionals to lead as well.

Because a number of physicians and diagnostic clinics primarily deal with adults, it is important that the age of the children served by the physicians and clinics be known.

Types of Evaluation Procedures

The traditional medical evaluation includes both the taking of a medical history and physical examination of the child. Both history-taking and examination are carried out with a number of different purposes. There is no one established format for these procedures, nor is an extremely exhaustive medical history necessary. History-taking can be directed toward the handicaps suspected. The examination can also take many forms and vary in length. The following descriptions are examples of these procedures.

The History

The medical history can serve a number of purposes. It is usually taken in chronological order. In the early part of the history one may look for evidence of insults to the developing organism, before birth, during delivery, after birth, and even within the early years of childhood. Many studies have sought to correlate these early events with later outcome, but the data are only statistical, and in very few cases can these early events be correlated with later handicapping conditions with absolute certainty. The other etiological factors are genetic in origin and are explored when the family medical history is taken. The history will be continued chronologically to inquire about significant medical illnesses that may influence the developing child and may represent potential or current conditions that could interfere with educational processes.

Along with the history of medical conditions, the physician will also take a developmental history, which can provide valuable information as to early deficits in developmental processes that may be the precursors of a current developmental disability (handicap). This early history is retrospective and depends upon the memory of the parents. Early motor developmental difficulties, such as failure to walk at the appropriate time, or failure to develop language according to established norms or at the appropriate time, may strongly indicate that handicapping conditions are likely.

The physician also inquires about the child's behavior at certain stages, in order to obtain valuable information as to the child's current behavioral status. Correlations between early behaviors and school behavior are sometimes quite strong.

In addition, the physician asks about the child's exposure to a school environment, starting with earliest pre-school experiences. If necessary, the child's learning and behavioral patterns can be followed year by year. Simultaneously, the environment in which the child is situated can be explored, so as to correlate development with the expectations of those around the child, together with his or her relationships with peers. Once again, the developmental process is such that early difficulties, such as prolonged reversals of letters or words, can be of significant help in understanding present conditions, when the aforementioned dysfunction has ceased to operate because of maturational processes that have occurred in the meantime.

The most relevant inquiry of all is with regard to the child's present status, both in school and in the home. Additionally, it is pertinent to inquire about the child's function in any or all environments, which can include outside activities such as shopping, going to religious services, playing with peers, and visiting relatives. It is also important to ascertain the nature of the environment in which the child is living as well as his or her behavior in both social activities and in homework.

The aim of this history is to provide a sum total of the child's experiences from conception to the present. Etiological factors are the least important because of their lack of relevance to the ultimate development of an individualized education plan. Developmental data is potentially more helpful in the current diagnosis, but there is the risk that inaccurate reporting by the parent may lead to misdiagnosis of the earlier situations. The most important part of the history is exploration of the child's current status.

The Examination

Examination should, ideally, consist of three parts. The first, and usually least rewarding part, is the general physical examination. This is fully relevant only when the handicapping condition involves other systems than the nervous system, and in many cases will have to be carried out by a specialist in the appropriate medical system involved. The only other reason for the general physical examination is to look for accompanying signs that might help diagnose the particular problem for which the child is being evaluated. In this respect there is a strong correlation between conditions of the skin and conditions of the nervous system; a very careful examination of the skin is an absolute requirement in all children who have handicapping conditions involving the nervous system.

The second part consists of a full examination of the nervous system designed to find, or more often to rule out, physical signs that are known to correlate with actual disease processes in the nervous system. A formal neurological examination for signs of disease is carried out simultaneously with the third part of the examination, which is the most relevant from the point of view of evaluating a child for a handicapping condition. This is a neurodevelopmental examination that looks at the nervous system to determine whether a particular system is functioning correctly for the age level of the child. For this reason the child must be evaluated through a series of tests that have been applied to children of different ages and for which there are established normal standards. These developmental neurological signs are commonly known as "soft" signs, a term first used by Clements and Peters (1962) in identifying some of the "equivocal" and "dubious" neurological signs considered to be associated with signs of a learning disability. Since then, many physicians have used the same signs from a developmental point of view, pointing out that these signs, which follow a developmental curve, are more likely to be present in younger children and less likely in older children. The original description, with a follow-up by Peters, Romine, and Dykman (1975), was mostly concerned with signs of motor dysfunction, but the same principle can be applied to all systems in the brain. For this reason it could be legitimate to consider the data from psychologists as representing neurological soft signs when psychological testing shows deviation from the norm for the age of the child. All examiners on the interdisciplinary team, when concerned with the processes of learning, are measuring the presence or absence of soft signs, which represent a deviation from the norm. In practice, the physician, as well as other members of the team, can also measure the child's deviation above the norm; such a deviation is not, of course, termed a soft sign, as the implication of the term is that it represents a developmental deficit.

The physician who is looking for soft signs may well carry his or her examination beyond the formal motor signs as first described and may also look at sensory areas. One important sensory measurement is of the child's awareness of left and right, which follows a developmental pattern. Specific testing of right-left orientation may correlate with problems in reversing letters and words in the classroom. This can be measured during the developmental examination.

The physician may also use tests of the brain's ability to process visual information as well as auditory information in addition to testing vision and hearing. In this respect he or she is overlapping with the areas of the psychologist, the speech pathologist, and the audiologist, and his or her final conclusions may be similar to their findings. This practice provides a further evaluation of the child through a different discipline, and the correlation of the two sets of data can be very important. One absolute requirement is that the physician must not use the same test that any of his or her colleagues use, because of the existence of test-retest problems if the same test is applied again too close in time to the first test. The same problem can exist for the psychologist and the speech pathologist if they both happen to use the same test battery.

One option available to the medical examiner is to carry out the examination prior to exploring the history or examining other data, so as not to be biased by the information given by the parent. The ultimate goal of this evaluation is *not* to produce a label for the child but to engender a diagnostic profile. The analogy that can be used here is to a jigsaw puzzle; a picture can be seen without necessarily having every piece in place, but sufficient pieces are needed to produce a clear picture. The picture in this case is how the child functions, and the basic rule is that the approach must be holistic. For this reason, all systems should be touched on and inquired into, if only to rule out associated conditions. For the prime handicapping condition more detail is needed, and no one professional on the team can accurately evaluate all aspects of it. The final diagnostic profile must be assembled by the whole team.

IMPLICATIONS FOR IEP DEVELOPMENT

As previously stated, the physician is less likely to be expert in the formalization of an individualized education plan and for that reason will rely upon other team members to utilize medical findings and translate them into formalized educational planning. It is doubtful whether the presence of the physician at the IEP meeting is of value. In most cases, those concerned with writing the IEP can call the physician to obtain additional information or an opinion in any area. In most cases, the final planning for the recommendations made by the physician will be channeled through a particular member of the school team, who may be the psychologist, physical therapist, occupational therapist, or special educator.

ISSUES, CONCERNS, AND RECOMMENDATIONS

Although the medical evaluation can cover the same ground as the evaluations by other members of the team, in most cases it is carried out at a remote site. The recommendations made by the physician will, in fact, resemble those made by educational therapists, but will be stated in different terms. The basic principle of utilizing brain function in any handicapping condition is that of using the stronger areas for day-to-day activity while endeavoring to remediate those areas of the brain that are functioning poorly. It is possible for the physician, on a neurodevelopmental basis, to make fairly specific recommendations in this respect. In some cases, the physician can recommend the use of a sign language interpreter as well as talking books and tape recorders. The physician can also sign an authorization form for the use of the talking book system funded by the Library of Congress.

Specific recommendations as to educational techniques to be used in weak areas are normally beyond the province of the physician. In fact, the value of a physician's recommendations is proportional to the degree of cooperation between physician and school systems, by which each learns from the other and establishes a common language. On the whole, the medical evaluation is probably most helpful in aiding other members of the team to make recommendations, with the requirement that the medical evaluation is put into terms that can be readily understood by the different disciplines represented on the team.

The best way for the physician to make recommendations is jointly with other members of the evaluation team, and not just in a written report following the evaluation. For this reason, the next step for the physician is to meet with as many of the members of the team as possible to discuss results of all evaluations and to consolidate the information. A "case conference" is built into the best medical systems, and should the medical evaluation be part of a team approach in a diagnostic clinic, it is vital that those working with the child in the educational facility be invited to this conference. It cannot be too strongly emphasized that sending reports to and fro is a very poor substitute for discussion.

Recommendations for the non-neurological handicapping conditions listed under "other health impaired" in the federal regulations may well need to be more medical than educational. The physician who is particularly expert in the area under consideration, whether it be chronic lung disease, congenital heart disease, or orthopedic problems, must take the lead in describing what activities the child may and may not participate in. With severe visual and hearing impairments, close coordination with the school system is necessary before a final disposition can be made. In these latter conditions and in severe emotional handicaps, it is clear that direct medical therapy will probably be needed. Medical therapy is, of course, within the province of the medical community and is in addition to any services needed from an educational point of view.

Indications for Laboratory Procedures

It will be noted that the section concerned with the actual examination of the child made no reference to laboratory procedures. If the physician is dealing with a suspected disease within the system, laboratory testing will, in most cases, be indicated. Physicians dealing with medical conditions other than the processes of behavior in learning may well need actual laboratory investigations to measure function or dysfunction in a system. They will be recommended and carried out by the appropriate specialist.

In the case of the nervous system, a considerable range of laboratory procedures are available. In most cases, these procedures are being utilized for the identification or exclusion of a disease process and for this reason are not relevant to most of the neurological handicapping conditions. In the majority of cases, no active disease element is present, and the most that such procedures can establish is that a condition was present in the past. This information is not only academic but in most cases is far less accurate than the clinical evaluation that has preceded it.

X-ray procedures are very easy to carry out but neither formal x-rays nor the CAT scan can do more than provide anatomical correlates. They do not show function. The electroencephalogram (EEG) shows electrical activity in the brain, and there are statistical correlations between certain EEG abnormalities and certain forms of brain dysfunctions, but the correlations are weak and cannot be applied to individual cases. Once again the clinical evaluation is infinitely more accurate in measuring function or dysfunction than the EEG. An EEG can occasionally be used to diagnose or, more likely, to rule out a seizure disturbance. Nevertheless, clinical judgment supersedes laboratory results.

Despite claims of finding correlations between conditions such as infantile autism and chemical abnormalities, there is no accepted biochemical abnormality that can be measured and used to diagnose these handicapping conditions. Chromosomal studies can be utilized to identify a small number of genetic disorders, of which Down's syndrome is the best known.

In most cases, clinical diagnosis will accurately precede the chromosomal confirmation. In a certain number of children, chromosomal abnormalities will be found that were not previously suspected, but the fact remains that no therapeutic or educational recommendations can be made as a result of finding the chromosomal abnormality. The sole reason for these procedures would be for providing genetic counseling to the family, if sufficient data are available, because the findings are irrelevant to the educational process. Only the accurate clinical evaluation by members of the diagnostic team can identify the educational needs of the handicapped child.

Terminology for Behavior Disorders

Another topic which should be discussed here relates to the terminology in use with children who exhibit behavioral problems. Classification of behavior disorders is continually changing and always under dispute, but there is a considerable difference between the behavioral diagnoses made in Public Law 94-142 and those commonly in use in the medical profession. For this reason, children whose behavioral disturbances interfere with their education may occasionally be labeled differently by the medical profession. An example of this is infantile autism, which was originally categorized by Public Law 94-142 as a severe emotional handicap at a time when the medical profession recognized it as a neurological problem and primarily a distortion of behavioral development. At that time, only a psychiatrist was supposed to be able to diagnose autism, and psychiatrists did not accept it as an emotional handicap. This discrepancy has now been remedied. Autism has been reclassified as "other health impaired."

The same problem arises with children who are diagnosed medically as having an attention deficit disorder. It is estimated that almost 5 per cent of children may show some signs of this dysfunction, which represents a developmental delay in paying attention. In a considerable number of these children, the deficit is severe enough to interfere significantly with learning, and such children may end up with medical rather than psychological recommendations. The physician will regard this condition as a neurological impairment and not an emotional problem. For this reason, if the child needs any special educational services, he or she would not be classified as severely emotionally handicapped by the medical team. Nevertheless, many of these children have to be diagnosed as seriously emotionally disturbed in order to receive special education and related services.

Public Law 94-142 does not consider health services provided by a physician to be related services. However, when a health service that can be provided by a non-physician is provided by a physician, a school district would be required to pay for this service, although only as much as it would cost when provided by a non-physician.

REFERENCES

Berlin, R. (1887). Eine besondere art von wortblindheit (dyslexie); Monograph. Wiesbaden: Veilag von J. F. Bergann.

Broca, P. (1865). Sur le siège de la faculté du langage articulé. *Bulletin of Social Anthropology, 6*, 337–393.

Clements, S. D., & Peters, J. E. (1962). Minimal brain dysfunction in the school age child (diagnosis and treatment). *Archives of General Psychiatry, 6*, 185.

Education of the Handicapped Regulations. (1985). 34 Code of Federal Regulations Part 300, Supplement 138.

Hinshelwood, H. (1895). Word blindness and visual memory. *Lancet, 2*, 1564–1570.

Peters, J. E., Romine, J. S., & Dykman, R. A. A special neurological examination of children with learning disabilities. *Developmental Medicine and Child Neurology, 17*, 63–78.

Wernicke, K. (1874). Der aphasische symptomencomplex. Eine Psychologische Studie auf Anatomischer Basis. Breslau: Cohn and Weigert.

Chapter 7

Occupational Therapy

Charlotte Exner

Occupational therapy (OT) is a health care profession that focuses on the assessment and treatment of children who have impairments of daily life functioning. Aspects of daily life functioning that are addressed by occupational therapists include activities of daily living (ADL), school and work skills, and play and leisure skills. The occupational therapist is concerned with factors that cause problems in the functional aspects of living. These factors can include motor, sensory and sensory integrative, cognitive/perceptual, psychological/emotional, and social components of functioning.

Overall, the occupational therapist is concerned with the problems that make the child more dependent or less functional than desirable or necessary. The focus of occupational therapy is to provide intervention that will allow the child to function optimally and to assume the most independent role in society possible. When complete independence and full employment are not feasible, the occupational therapist aids the child in attaining competence in as many skills as possible.

DEFINITION OF OCCUPATIONAL THERAPY

Public Law 94-142 provides the following definition of occupational therapy: it "includes: (1) improving, developing, or restoring functions impaired or lost through illness, injury, or deprivation; (2) improving ability to perform tasks for independent functioning when functions are impaired or lost; and (3) preventing, through early intervention, initial or further impairment or loss of function" (Education of the Handicapped Regulations, 1985).

Occupational therapists (OTs) and occupational therapy assistants (OTAs) work with individuals and groups of people who have acute or chronic problems or who show potential for having such problems. Services are provided to occupational therapy consumers in educational, medical, and community settings, according to the needs of these consumers. Occupational therapists work closely with other professionals such as physical therapists, speech and language pathologists, nurses, physicians, nutritionists, psychologists, social workers, and educators (depending upon the type of setting) in order to provide an optimal and comprehensive program for the individual.

RELATIONSHIP TO SPECIAL EDUCATION

"As a related service, occupational therapy is provided to enhance students' abilities to adapt to and function in educational programs" (Gilfoyle and Farace, 1981). The focus of occupational therapy in this type of setting is to provide children with services designed to assist them in benefitting optimally from the learning opportunities provided by the educational program. Occupational therapy, with its focus on optimal functioning in daily life tasks, often plays an important role in helping the child to function in the least restrictive environment.

Role of the Therapist

Gilfoyle and Farace (1981) state that the roles of the occupational therapist in the school setting include evaluation of children, participation in the individualized education program (IEP) process, and implementation of treatment. In addition, they consult with parents, teachers, and other professionals regarding the child's abilities and disabilities and any appropriate precautions and limitations for the child. Thus, the occupational therapist has responsibility for providing services to children as well as for interacting with other professionals. Performance of related administrative duties, such as management and supervision of the occupational therapy program, is also an important part of most therapists' role.

The most common reasons for referral to occupational therapy are: difficulty in the fine motor area (e.g., grasping, using both hands, writing and cutting with scissors); obvious perceptual or perceptual motor problems; general clumsiness; positioning problems and the need for adaptive equipment for physically handicapped children; difficulty with chewing or swallowing; and inability to effectively eat independently. The occupational therapist needs to focus the evaluation and treatment of the child toward the reason for referral, although treatment for underlying problems creating the more obvious dysfunctions is often necessary.

Candidates for Therapy

Children who are most often treated by occupational therapists are those whose functioning in school, work, and activities of daily living is not in line with their cognitive development or who are at risk of losing functional abilities and skills. Today, infants and young children who are noted to be at "high risk" for sensory or motor problems are typically referred to occupational therapy for at least a screening before specific problems are ruled out. In addition to this high-risk group, school children with the following diagnoses are most commonly seen by occupational therapists for evaluation or treatment:

Cerebral palsy and other conditions affecting central nervous system functioning

Meningomyelocele (spina bifida)

Mental retardation—especially if associated motor, sensory, or perceptual deficits are present or if the child engages in self-injurious behaviors

Autism

Traumatic injuries, such as of the head or spinal cord (after medical healing)

Sensory impairments—visual or hearing

Learning disability—especially if associated with clumsiness, balance problems, poor coordination, perceptual-motor problems, or poor handwriting

Emotional disturbances

Degenerative disorders, such as muscular dystrophy

Juvenile rheumatoid arthritis

Evaluation of Children

Specific areas that occupational therapists address in the evaluation of children who are in school programs are:

Activities of daily living—eating (both oral motor and independent eating skills), dressing, personal hygiene, and community living skills.

School and work skills—writing, coloring, drawing, using scissors and other classroom tools; managing books and papers; participating in nonacademic areas such as art, music, and physical education; sitting effectively in the classroom; and using mobility for interaction with materials and other children. Prevocational and vocational skills are typically addressed in older children.

Play, leisure, and recreation skills—participating in art, music, physical education classes and playing with other children at recess and lunch times.

If problems in these areas are reported or observed, the occupational therapist continues the evaluation by assessing the child in some or all of the
following areas:

Motor functioning—fine motor and gross motor skills and aspects of the
child's neuromotor functioning that provide the foundation for motor skills.

Sensory and sensory integration functioning—sensory assessment, which
involves the child's awareness of input through touch, joint movement, and
body position and movement, and ability to make use of visual abilities.
Sensory integration (SI) evaluation specifically addresses the child's ability
to combine input from a variety of senses so as to develop the ability to
control the body against gravity (postural control); to feel comfortable with
movement (postural security); to use both sides of the body together effectively (bilateral integration); to know the various parts of one's body and
how they relate to one another (body scheme); to respond to touch from
others appropriately (tactile system integration); and to carry out activities
that involve sequences of actions (motor planning).

Cognitive and perceptual functioning—the ability to attend to tasks; to show
appropriate judgment; to make decisions; to follow orderly sequences for
task completion; to see relationships among various objects; to remember
relationships among objects; and to use perceptual-motor skills.

Psychological and emotional functioning—frustration tolerance, methods for
dealing with anxiety and failures, dependence on others, self-concept and
self-esteem. This area is usually addressed in conjunction with one of the
other areas.

Social functioning—ability to work effectively with others; to cooperate;
to communicate ideas and needs; and to obtain satisfaction from interactions with others. This area is usually addressed in conjunction with one of
the other areas.

Providing Services (Therapy)

Occupational therapists treat children using a variety of techniques. Treatment may include methods for improving the quality of motor functioning
or increasing motor skills, sensory integration activities, perceptual-motor
activities, play activities, simulated school or work tasks, and intervention
for self-care or other tasks of daily living. The therapist may also develop
and teach the child how to use adaptive equipment and compensatory
strategies to accomplish specific tasks. Positioning adaptations, in order to
view materials, the teacher, and other children as well as to perform tasks
such as writing, eating, and dressing more effectively are a priority area for
many children.

Occupational therapists also make splints for some physically disabled children for the purpose of preventing arm and hand deformities and optimizing hand function. Intervention with children may focus primarily upon prevention of future problems or delays, remediation of current problems and delays, or compensations for current problems so that the child can perform functional skills in the near future.

Cooperation with Teachers

Although the occupational therapist collaborates with the child's teacher and others in developing the child's IEP plan, on-going collaboration is essential for optimal results. The therapist and the teacher need to share information about their perspectives on the child's problems and assets. Attention to effective integration of therapeutic activities into classroom activities is needed for mildly affected children who are mainstreamed (placed in the regular school program with support personnel and services). In these situations, both the teacher and the therapist need to carefully divide the typical classroom activities into those that need extensive modification and those that could be modified slightly to allow the child to gain other benefits.

With children who are more severely handicapped, integration of therapeutic principles into classroom activities is expected and somewhat more easily accomplished. Regardless of the severity of the child's problems, the therapist needs to have regular informal as well as formal meetings with the teacher in order to discuss the child's progress as well as any difficulties with suggested techniques. In some cases, teachers and therapists collaborate on data collection for more objective monitoring of a child's progress. Responsibility for all aspects of program implementation needs to be clearly specified, so that teachers and therapists can minimize role confusion and misunderstandings (Stephens, 1985). In addition, periodic discussion of each person's priorities for the child and key strategies being used to attain these are helpful.

Administrative Responsibility

Another type of responsibility of occupational therapists that affects their involvement in the educational process is in the area of administration. As identified by the American Occupational Therapy Association (1980), these duties include development and periodic review of the occupational therapy program provided to children in the school district, maintenance of records, preparation and monitoring of budgets, knowledge of community resources, and maintenance and enhancement of each therapist's competency through attendance at professional meetings, consultation with experts in various practice areas, and involvement in continuing education.

Qualifications of Occupational Therapists and Occupational Therapy Assistants

An occupational therapist holds a bachelor's degree or a master's degree in occupational therapy from a program accredited by the American Medical Association and the American Occupational Therapy Association. The academic program addresses medical, physical, psychological, and social aspects of function and dysfunction. Traditionally, occupational therapy educational programs emphasized the medical model, which is concerned with illness and dysfunction; however, the public schools employ the concept of learning, not of sickness and wellness (Stephens, 1985). Recently with increasing numbers of occupational therapists being employed by school systems, university academic programs have begun to place more emphasis on teaching students about educational models of service delivery.

As part of their training, occupational therapists complete a minimum of six months of full-time field work experience in approved clinical settings. Three months are typically spent in a psychosocial (mental health) setting and three months in a physical disabilities setting. Some students pursue additional pediatric training. Students are generally oriented toward acute and chronic problems seen in individuals of various ages through these field work experiences and through other clinical experiences during their academic programs.

At the conclusion of the academic course work and the field work experiences, all occupational therapy students take a national certification examination. An individual who has successfully passed the examination is eligible to use the title Occupational Therapist, Registered (OTR). Many states now also require occupational therapists to be licensed in order to practice. All of the states that require licensure use the national standards set by the American Occupational Therapy Association and the same national certifying examination scores. Licensure boards (boards of occupational therapy practice) in some states require occupational therapists to meet certain continuing competency requirements in order to renew their licenses yearly. These competency requirements typically consist of evidence of participation in relevant continuing education experiences. Most occupational therapists also maintain their certification with the American Occupational Therapy Association. Some state and local boards of education have additional requirements for the therapists they employ.

The responsibilities of occupational therapists and occupational therapy assistants are somewhat different. An occupational therapist is responsible for evaluation, treatment planning, treatment implementation, design and construction of some adaptive equipment, and administrative tasks, including supervision of certain personnel. Occupational therapy assistants are supervised by occupational therapists. An occupational therapy assistant is primarily responsible for treatment implementation and construction of some types of adaptive equipment. The occupational therapy assistant also notes changes in a child's status and modifies a child's program in response to these changes, usually in collaboration with the supervising occupational therapist.

Occupational therapy assistant programs must be approved by the American Occupational Therapy Association. These are typically one to two year programs from which the student earns an associate degree. The focus of these programs is similar to that of the occupational therapy programs. OTA students also have various clinical experiences during their academic work and complete two to three months of full-time clinical work after completing their academic courses. They must also pass a national examination. Upon completion of the examination, they are certified by the American Occupational Therapy Association and may use the initials COTA. Some states require OT assistants to be licensed.

OPTIONS IN SERVICE DELIVERY MODELS

Occupational therapy treatment may be carried out in a separate occupational therapy room, in the child's classroom, in other settings in the school (depending upon the needs of the child), or in the child's home. Most children benefit from intervention in a combination of these settings, so that all key individuals are aware of the child's program and progress and can give input for program adjustment. Using a variety of settings is also helpful for generalization of new skills.

The two basic types of occupational therapy service models are direct services and indirect services. Most occupational therapists provide both. Evaluation and participation in program design for children are included in both models. Also, in both models the occupational therapist has the responsibility of educating those involved with the child about particular problems that fall under the scope of occupational therapy practice. The service models may include home program recommendations for the child, as well as other types of programming.

Children may receive direct or indirect services from an occupational therapist, regardless of their type of school placement. Children who are mainstreamed are more likely to receive services from an itinerant therapist (one who travels to many schools) than children who are in self-contained classrooms where they are taught by the same teacher during the entire school day, or in schools primarily for children receiving total special education programs. Often, the latter type of school has at least one school-based occupational therapist.

Direct Services

Direct service implies that the therapist works directly with the child on either an individual or a group basis (Clark and Allen, 1985; Stephens, 1985). In direct service, the occupational therapist or the occupational therapy assistant is held accountable for the outcome of the treatment program (Clark and Allen, 1985). Children who are treated with direct services generally receive occupational therapy treatment at least once a week (Stephens, 1985), with some children receiving treatment up to five times a week; the most typical frequency is twice a week. Direct services include screening, evaluation, and treatment planning for occupational therapy programs as well as total IEP plans, treatment implementation, re-evaluation, and, ultimately, discharge planning (American Occupational Therapy Association, 1980).

Indirect Services

Indirect services include both services to children and administrative responsibilities. Indirect services provided to children are currently divided into two main categories, monitoring and consultation (Clark and Allen, 1985). In both categories, the therapist usually evaluates the child and determines the services the child needs.

When *monitoring* a child, the therapist has decided that the child can receive the necessary intervention from a person other than the occupational therapist (Clark and Allen, 1985). In this case, the therapist develops an intervention plan and trains others to implement it. Those who may be trained to implement such a program include the classroom teacher, physical education teacher, adaptive physical education specialist, and resource teachers who specialize in reading or writing. The therapist monitors the child and the program, making changes as needed, and is ultimately responsible for the program's effectiveness (Clark and Allen, 1980). Children who are being monitored by the occupational therapist usually meet with the primary program implementer approximately once a week or once every two weeks. The precaution one must keep in mind about the monitoring system is that not all children are appropriate for this service model, though it initially may seem appealing to those responsible for ensuring that all children who need to see an occupational therapist do so. Some children need the expertise of the occupational therapist in their treatment program. As Langdon and Langdon (1983) note, "only a therapist may conduct therapeutic activities with a student. . . . Conduct of supplemental activities by personnel other than the occupational therapist must be closely monitored by the therapist to ensure proper application of procedures and adherence to necessary precautions."

Consultation is the other category of indirect service. The therapist typically makes some type of assessment of the child, although this may be less complete than the evaluation of other types of service delivery. The occupational therapist then provides recommendations to the person who referred the child. Usually, contact is made on a monthly basis at most and may actually occur only when changes are made in the child's status (for example, when the child is changed to a new classroom, is faced with new architectural barriers, or needs new equipment). In some cases a therapist is consulted about an individual child only once. In this type of professional relationship the occupational therapist is not responsible for the implementation of the recommendations about the child (Clark and Allen, 1985). An occupational therapist may consult with a child's classroom teacher, resource teacher, art or music teacher, speech therapist, physical therapist, or physician.

Occupational therapists may also be asked to consult with staff about issues affecting a number of students, such as architectural barriers, learning materials, and physical education activities. They may also give in-service presentations to other professionals and to parents, consult with directors of other programs a child is part of, and participate in specific IEP meetings at the request of the school administration (American Occupational Therapy Association, 1980).

IMPLICATIONS FOR IEP DEVELOPMENT

Assessment

Clark and Allen (1985) state that the first three steps of the occupational therapist's assessment of the child are to document the child's present functioning, to delineate the child's problems, and to determine the child's potential for change and progress. In order to perform these steps, the therapist must be knowledgeable about standardized and nonstandardized tests appropriate for children with developmental problems, and must be able to integrate the findings of all the measures used.

Using this information, the occupational therapist defines the child's strengths (assets) and weaknesses (problem areas) and makes a determination about the child's potential for improvement as well as the approximate length of time needed to accomplish certain goals. Assets, which may contribute to expectations that goals have a high likelihood of being met more quickly in some children than others, include the following:

1. Child variables—motivation to improve, a reasonable attention span, obvious readiness for attaining a skill, and fewer factors contributing to the problem.
2. Adult (parent, teacher) variables—willingness to invest time in the child's program, understanding of the reasons for the child's problems, strong desire for the child to accomplish the skill, and rapport with the child.
3. Environmental variables—availability of needed equipment and materials at home and school, funding for special equipment needed, availability of appropriate space for treatment (quiet, spacious enough to allow for program implementation), and sufficient time to treat the child (in terms of both the child's schedule and the therapist's schedule).

The therapist documents the occupational therapy evaluation findings for the child's file (Stephens, 1985) and determines the need for occupational therapy services on the basis of the outcome of the evaluation. However, an occupational therapy program may be provided only after written consent is received from the child's parents or legal guardian (Stephens, 1985; Langdon and Langdon, 1983). Some school systems require parental consent for an occupational therapy evaluation.

An IEP for the child who has been referred to occupational therapy contains several types of input from the therapist.

Goals and Objectives

After the key points from the evaluation are noted, goals and objectives for the child are specified. Usually, the intention of the goals is that they will be accomplished in one year. These goals may be conceived of as being short-term or long-term goals for a particular child, based on the severity of the child's disability. For example, a more severely handicapped child may be expected to require intervention for several years, and each yearly goal may actually be a step toward a larger goal to be met three to five years later. In contrast, a one-year goal for a more mildly impaired child may actually represent the endpoint of therapy for that child. Typically, an IEP for a child who needs occupational therapy has one or more goals that will be addressed by the occupational therapist. Occupational therapy goals should complement the educational performance goals for that student (Langdon and Langdon, 1983). In contrast to goals, objectives are written in more specific and measurable terms. They represent the steps to accomplishing the goals. The anticipated grading of the intervention program is often evident in the description of the objectives.

Specific Services to Be Provided, Including Extent

Several other components are included in children's IEP plans. After identification of goals and objectives, the methods to be used in working toward the objectives are specified. Methods may include such approaches as neurodevelopmental treatment (handling and positioning) for gross, fine, and oral motor problems, sensory integration treatment, and use of graded activities for development of ADL skills. At this point, the decision regarding individual versus group treatment must be made. Whereas some children need one-to-one intervention, because of their need for close monitoring of the quality of their performance or because of privacy issues, other children benefit from group treatment. Social interaction with peers can be very useful in treatment, and some children are inspired to work toward more independence when given peer support. Certain social-emotional goals may be addressed best through group interaction, rather than in one-to-one interaction between the child and the therapist. Groups of two to three students are often the most appropriate size to work with (Langdon and Langdon, 1983).

The responsibilities of all team members for implementation of the child's IEP are specified. For the occupational therapist, this identification of responsibilities includes the frequency of occupational therapy, the length of the treatment sessions, the beginning date of therapy, and the expected total duration of treatment (Stephens, 1985). Langdon and Langdon (1983) suggest that the minimum length of an occupational therapy treatment session be 30 to 40 minutes, given the need for equipment preparation and documentation as well as treatment of the child. Preferably, the children's treatment sessions can be coordinated with their schedules for classes at school.

Several factors contribute to the occupational therapist's decision regarding whether or not, how often, and how long to treat a child. The key factors are the therapist's judgment about the significance of the problem(s) to the child's educational functioning and how likely the problem is to respond to treatment. Particular problem areas that are high priority include:

difficult physical management of the child in the classroom
fine motor problems that interfere with classroom functioning
skills needed to be mainstreamed or to remain in a regular class placement
lack of adequate, upright body positioning or problems with the child's
    adaptive equipment
lack of independence in activities of daily living or wheelchair mobility in a
    child who shows strong evidence of potential in these areas
oral motor functioning that impairs the child's ability to take in adequate
    food or liquid.

Other factors will also influence the therapist's decision regarding the need for occupational therapy. For example, a child who has had no prior treatment is often considered to be more likely to show greater initial progress in therapy than a child who has had continual treatment over a number of years. Age of the child is a factor in many therapists' treatment decisions, with younger children receiving priority for services (Gilfoyle and Hays, 1981; Stephens, 1985). Stephens (1985) has a system by which therapists may determine a child's degree of need for therapy. In this system the therapist assigns points to various factors believed to contribute to successful responses to treatment, and subtracts points for factors believed to interfere with therapy outcome. Although some therapists and administrators give priority for treatment to severely handicapped children and keep these children on direct therapy for a number of years, others believe that these children may attain adequate educational benefits from monitoring and consultative services. Continuous, long-term therapy may not be necessary for all of these children, though they may need direct services periodically.

Less severely affected children, including some learning-disabled children, often receive fewer services than more severely handicapped children. However, the former typically have significant potential for functional improvement when given direct occupational therapy services, and may need these services for much shorter times than children with more severe disabilities.

Factors not directly related to the individual child's status may also influence the decision about frequency and duration of treatment. They include the therapist's and the child's schedules, the therapist's role in the school system (for example, whether itinerant or not, documentation requirements, administrative responsibilities, consultations expected), and the number of hours the child is in school and the number of hours the therapist provides services (Gilfoyle and Hays, 1981). The presence of an occupational therapy assistant will also affect the therapist's decisions regarding delivery of treatment services.

Another issue affecting provision of some occupational therapy services is the need for physician referral. Some states have regulations that require an occupational therapist to have a physician's referral in order to evaluate and treat a child, and other states do not. However, physician input may be extremely helpful when assessing the child, determining the child's problems, developing treatment goals, and planning treatment, including precautions for treatment activities. In addition, therapists typically find that keeping the child's physician apprised of the child's progress in therapy promotes an enhanced professional relationship.

Criteria and Evaluation of Progress

The IEP contains methods for measuring the child's progress or lack of progress. Using these methods for determining whether the goals have been met, and any other testing or interviews deemed necessary, the therapist re-evaluates the child at least yearly. After this re-evaluation, the therapist determines the need for further occupational therapy services, the goal(s) of these services, and appropriate frequency. The standard typically used for decreasing frequency of services, changing a child from direct to indirect services, or discontinuing therapy for a specific child is that the therapy goals have been accomplished or the child has recently plateaued—that is, has shown no obvious functional improvement (American Occupational Therapy Association, 1980; Clark and Allen, 1985). Many times the child's treatment is changed from direct services to monitoring, then to consultation, as a way of ensuring that the child maintains important skills. Children may also be moved to more intensive services if these services are warranted.

ISSUES, CONCERNS, AND RECOMMENDATIONS

Case Overload

One of the major issues facing occupational therapists in the school system is how to provide services effectively for all the children who need therapy. Occupational therapists are often expected to see large numbers of children and to use primarily consultation and monitoring rather than direct treatment. Some therapists carry caseloads of more than 100 students, and some cover students in several school districts, in the course of one week. To address these issues, the Task Force on School System Issues, appointed by the American Occupational Therapy Association, is in the process of developing guidelines for occupational therapist caseloads. The guidelines will take into account travel time between schools, necessary time for administrative duties, number of evaluations expected weekly, and levels of service needed by the children on the therapist's caseload. Stephens (1985) also suggests a mechanism for computing the number of students, based on various levels of service, that a therapist may be able to treat.

Many therapists try to solve their "case overload" by treating children less frequently than desirable for the children's needs. When this occurs, children may show less benefit from therapy than they could. The other strategy commonly used is to provide direct services to more severely handicapped children and fewer (or no) direct services to mildly impaired children. In some cases, this arrangement is quite unfortunate, as children with mild disabilities often have greater potential for being mainstreamed, for remaining mainstreamed, for vocational independence, and for independent living. They are also likely to benefit enough from therapy that their occupational therapy intervention can be reduced to a monitoring or consultant level much sooner than children with more severe disabilities. This criticism is not meant to imply that severely handicapped children do not need occupational therapy services; they do, and they typically need direct services. However, mildly involved children also need and benefit from such services.

Determining Intensity of Service

An issue related to level of intervention for children is the importance of varying service intensity to best meet the needs of the child. Children with motor or sensorimotor problems often receive therapy once or twice a week throughout the school year. Because of the complexity of their problems, and because these children typically have problems that interfere with their learning abilities and memory skills, intervention on a more intensive, short-term basis may be particularly helpful. A child may benefit more from intensive therapy (four times a week) for 3 months than from less intensive therapy (twice a week) for 6 months. If a child were to receive intensive therapy for a portion of the school year, perhaps the child could be placed on a monitoring system for other months of the year. This system of service delivery would be particularly dependent upon cooperation from the school administration and from the child's classroom teacher, who would have an especially important role in program implementation while the child was being monitored by the occupational therapist.

Relationship with Classroom Teachers

Ottenbacher (1982) discusses issues that may influence the relationship between the occupational therapist and the child's teacher. He suggests that educators and therapists often approach a child from different perspectives, using different models for understanding the child's needs. Occupational therapists are likely to use a process approach, emphasizing *why* the child is having difficulty and using strategies that are designed to remediate the cause(s) of the child's problem. Ottenbacher notes that educators are more likely to use a task analysis approach, which relies more on teaching the child steps of a task and using remedial strategies when necessary. Much less stress is placed on ameliorating the cause of the problems. Such differences in perspectives may cause some controversy or misunderstanding between the therapist and the educator. However, this is not necessary if all professionals involved recognize the benefits of alternative approaches and the potential for combining approaches to effectively intervene with a particular child (Ottenbacher, 1982).

Similar issues apply to the collaboration necessary between regular classroom teachers and occupational therapists for effective mainstreaming of physically handicapped students into the regular education classrooms. Kinnealey and Morse (1979) describe a successful program for mainstreaming preschool and elementary school age children with diagnoses of cerebral palsy, spina bifida, and other disabilities. This program had a coordinator who maintained contact with the ·therapists, the social worker, and the children's parents. In addition, the coordinator observed the children in their school placements and intervened as soon as problems began to arise. Occupational therapists and other team members provided in-service presentations for the children's teachers to facilitate their understanding of specific problems and therapeutic intervention strategies. Such programs suggest the importance of close contact between professionals, such as occupational therapists and teachers, so that children can be placed *and* be successful in the least restrictive environment. Concerns about the child's problems may make some teachers reluctant to have children with disabilities in their classrooms. By sharing information and making suggestions for adaptation strategies, the occupational therapist can help make mainstreaming successful for all.

Availability of Resources

Another issue confronting occupational therapists is availability of special equipment that would optimize mainstreaming of some children or allow other children to reach a higher level of functioning. For example, funding for adaptive positioning equipment is often quite limited. Many severely disabled children would benefit from having power wheelchairs so that they could have more independence and greater ability to interact with peers, as other children do at school. Although such equipment may not be within the funding scope of all schools, the occupational therapist also may not have time available (owing to caseload constraints) to pursue other avenues of equipment funding. When this is the case, children who could be much more independent, and in some cases could be mainstreamed, are not. Therefore, funding for school-related equipment and time for therapists to pursue community resources for equipment funding so children can function more optimally in school continue to be problems.

A related problem is in regard to space and equipment. These resources may not be available for some types of occupational therapy services, particularly for therapists who work in more than one school. For example, therapists need various testing materials, particularly new ones as they become available, for evaluation of children. Supplies such as adapted writing tools, splinting materials, dycem, and specific treatment materials may not be available to therapists in all school districts. Related to this is the need for materials to use in adaptive equipment construction. Therapists also need to have access to a specialist in adaptive equipment construction and modification in order to accommodate children who outgrow their equipment or whose postural requirements change.

Continuing Education

The final pervasive influence on quality delivery of occupational therapy services in the school system is related to opportunities for continuing education for therapists. Occupational therapists, like other professionals, need opportunities to share knowledge with one another. One answer may be to have an occupational therapist consultant who could provide in-service training and specific recommendations for treatment of individual children. In addition, opportunities for peer group meetings among therapists in a school system or between school systems could be arranged. Another option may be to schedule workshops for therapists on days that coincide with teachers' professional days.

REFERENCES

American Occupational Therapy Association. (1980). Standards of practice for occupational therapy in schools. *American Journal of Occupational Therapy, 34*(13), 900–905.

Clark, P. N. & Allen, A. S. (1985). The role of occupational therapy in pediatrics. In P. N. Clark & A. S. Allen (Eds.), *Occupational therapy for children* (pp. 2-9). St. Louis: The C. V. Mosby Co.

Education of the Handicapped Regulations. (1985). 34 Code of Federal Regulations Part 300, Supplement 138.

Gilfoyle, E., & Farace, J. (1981). The role of occupational therapy as an education-related service. *American Journal of Occupational Therapy, 35*(12), 811.

Gilfoyle, E. M. (ed.), & Hays, C. (coordinator). (1981). Sample job description: Occupational therapist in public school facilities. In *Training: Occupational therapy educational management in schools. Vol. 1* (module 2, appendix D, pp. 52–54). Rockville, MD: American Occupational Therapy Association.

Kinnealey, M., & Morse, A. B. (1979). Educational mainstreaming of physically handicapped children. *American Journal of Occupational Therapy, 33*(6), 365–372.

Langdon, H. J. U., & Langdon, L. L. (1983). *Initiating occupational therapy programs within the public school systems: A guide for occupational therapists and public school administrators.* Thorofare, NJ: Charles B. Slack, Inc.

Ottenbacher, K. (1982). Occupational therapy and special education: Some issues and concerns related to Public Law 94-142. *American Journal of Occupational Therapy, 36*(2), 81–84.

Stephens, L. C. (1985). Occupational therapy in the school system. In P. N. Clark & A. S. Allen (Eds.), *Occupational therapy for children* (pp. 471–489). St. Louis: The C. V. Mosby Co.

Chapter 8

Parent Counseling and Training

Thelma L. Blumberg

Parent training may be described as a learning activity for parents who wish to improve relationships with their children. Interestingly enough, the idea is not really new, as the first group parent meeting in this country reportedly was held in Portland, Maine, in 1815. Yet, prior to the nineteenth century, child care information was entirely inspired by European models (Croake and Glover, 1977).

At the same time, formal parent counseling, as it relates to special education, is a twentieth century development. It may be described briefly as a helping process for solving human and family problems. The goals of counseling as they apply to parents of handicapped children may be equated with goals for anyone experiencing problems or coping with stress (Suran and Rizzo, 1979).

DEFINITION OF PARENT COUNSELING AND TRAINING

Parent counseling and training, as defined by Public Law 94-142, is assistance given to parents for understanding the special needs of their handicapped child. The law requires also that parents be provided with information about child development. Parent counseling and training, furthermore, is listed among those related services that may be required by a handicapped child in order to benefit from special education. The law specifies that these services be provided by qualified social workers, psychologists, guidance counselors, or other qualified personnel (Education of the Handicapped Regulations, 1985).

RELATIONSHIP TO SPECIAL EDUCATION

When we relate the effects of family needs to special education, we must consider three factors. First, the school and the family, needless to say, are intimately interrelated and reciprocally affect each other; second, the parents of handicapped children are frequently emotionally drained and often suffer from financial hardships, so that it is not at all surprising that stress and academic failure in school increase with these strains within the family; third, if we recognize that the family is the most powerful agent of change in the life of a child, it is impossible to ignore the dynamics within the family (Van Osdol and Shane, 1982).

It is interesting to note that over the past 20 years, there has been a change from an unofficial taboo to official endorsement of parent involvement in the education of their children. In fact, it has been strongly suggested that parent involvement has positive effects on the academic performance of children (Shapero and Forbes, 1981). Evidence also suggests that early involvement with other parents of handicapped children in programs designed to increase parental knowledge of both their children's disabilities and the educational options serves to reduce the negative impact that the handicapped condition has on the family (Kramer, 1985).

ELIGIBILITY FOR RELATED SERVICE PROVISION

Many professionals strongly advocate that servicing the special needs of parents of handicapped children promotes an economical use of school resources. Many arguments and observations elucidate and support this contention. Parents can never be fully prepared for the birth of a handicapped child. One parent described the shock and depersonalization of having a deaf child in these terms: "I was like a character in a play. And I could see myself acting a role. I asked questions and nodded. But I don't recall anything said. All I really wanted to do was go somewhere and hide" (Luterman, 1979). Often, the sheer mechanics of caring for a handicapped child create chronic fatigue, depression, and a sense of helplessness, causing a weakening of parents' confidence and decision making skills (Murray, 1985). Furthermore, instead of becoming more self-sufficient, some handicapped children require increasing time and energy with passing years. The prolonged interference with parents' personal freedom can lead to poor physical and mental health (Harris and Fong, 1985).

The child's natural environment is considered the best place to begin when striving to change behaviors. This reasoning leads to the home, and to the retraining of parents, which is usually desirable, and often absolutely necessary (O'dell, 1974).

The general public and even teachers and other professionals are not always positive in their attitudes toward the handicapped. In fact, handicapped children are often at risk for eliciting negative reactions such as pity, rejection, and taunting. The combined efforts of the counselor, the home, and the school may be necessary to counteract the difficulties faced by the child (Pfeiffer, 1980).

OPTIONS IN SERVICE DELIVERY MODELS

Providing parent counseling in the schools may have a variety of approaches. The emergence of innumerable books, programs, and audio and video tapes, along with a host of other tools for use with parent counseling and training, appears to be a vast and growing enterprise. Thus, space here permits only brief descriptions of some of the options available.

Parent Education

Parents of handicapped children, needless to say, may benefit from the same formal parent education programs that are offered to parents of non-handicapped children. Topics may comprise the developmental expectations of children in terms of gross motor, fine motor, language, self-help and cognitive areas, as they pertain to the infant, early childhood, the play age, school age, adolescent, and young adult. Additional topics are: information about specific disabilities; educational options; developing children's self-concept; sibling rivalry; getting the most out of time spent with children; children's allowances; and effective management of family routines.

Parent Training

Of the many strategies for teaching better parenting techniques, the three most popular are Systematic Training for Effective Parenting (STEP), Parent Effectiveness Training (PET), and behavioral management.

   The STEP program, published in 1976 and revised in 1983, is based on the theory and writings of Alfred Adler. The primary aims are to help parents understand the purpose of their children's behavior. Importance is also placed on teaching parents to guide their children toward responsibility and participation within the family group. The PET program, published in 1970, is based on the teachings of Carl Rogers and trains parents in listening techniques, communication skills, and child-parent problem-solving. Both programs include lectures, readings, role playing, demonstrations, and homework assignments, and both assume that there can be a better relationship between parents and children. Both, in addition, advocate more democratic methods of child-rearing, oppose authoritarian control, and favor the principle of mutual respect in parent-child relationships (Croake and Glover, 1977). Although the use of these programs has been widespread, it should be noted that there has been no substantial demonstration that they actually improve family relationships (Kramer, 1985).

At the same time, behavior management techniques (Becker, 1971; Patterson, 1971) have been found to produce positive changes in behavior and attitudes of both children and parents. There are two major approaches to teaching behavior management. The first consists of examination of the theoretical issues, or the universal rules of behavior, that affect common daily interactions: how behaviors are learned through reinforcement, modeling, and shaping; when and how to use reinforcement; how inappropriate behaviors can be eliminated; and rules for effective punishment. Examination of these principles reveals some surprising facts: (1) many unacceptable behaviors of children are actually taught by parents, usually accidentally; (2) even those unacceptable behaviors that have been ongoing for a very long time can be changed; (3) it is common practice for family members to complicate relationships with other family members by assigning complex and inaccurate motives to their behavior; (4) merely observing and defining a specific unacceptable behavior and then separating it from the child can, by itself, produce positive effects.

The second approach to teaching behavior management techniques involves the study and application of the actual behavior skills, such as defining, counting, and graphing frequencies of behavior, and applying consequences that will increase or decrease the frequencies of behaviors. These techniques have proved to be highly effective for reducing deviant, self-destructive, and aggressive behaviors as well as for improving communication skills. Along with drastic behavior changes, it is not unusual to see positive side effects such as better interpersonal relationships, enhanced self-concept, and increased productivity.

Parent Discussion Groups

Discussion with other parents may be both therapeutic and informative. Sessions often deal with such topics as sharing information about special techniques that have proved successful for specific disabilities, learning how other parents cope with similar situations, and generally airing concerns. The format for these meetings may be structured lectures, parent panel discussion, or exchange of views by interest groups.

Parent Counseling

Helping Through Periods of Stress

It is quite common to hear that some parents of handicapped children may be described as "defensive," "quarrelsome," or even "manipulative." But one must never lose sight of the fact that what each of these parents is really trying to say is, "I hurt inside; please help me!"

Blumberg (1985) describes some challenges that a counselor may face when meeting these parents. For one thing, many of the parents seen have children with low-incidence disabilities, and it becomes impossible to generalize problems from one client to another.

The counselor may erroneously anticipate that the parent is responsible in some way for the child's problem or, at the very least, that parenting skills are poor. Counselors become impatient with parents who fail to face the full reality of a child's disability immediately. In some instances it may serve no useful purpose, and in effect may be cruel, to demand total acceptance of severe trauma that could be swallowed more easily in small doses. Some of the parents seen have children with multiple physical and mental disabilities, making it appear as though a picture of despair on the part of the counselor is the only recourse. Professionals often mistakenly assume that the guilt feelings held by these parents should be the primary and immediate concern in counseling. In doing so, they overlook the fact that what they mistake for feelings of guilt may really be desperate cries for useful and immediate help for the problem child, the siblings, or simple daily management.

In truth, there is often no way that a counselor may know the parental stage of stress, or the immediate needs, without first seeking more information. Thus it is vital that open-ended questions be asked, such as, "Where do you need help most?" "What is the most difficult aspect of all of this for you, your child, or your family?" or simply "How can I help you?"

Sometimes a parent may benefit from just the right push to keep going and may welcome comments such as "It *is* possible for you to be happy again!" or "Yes, you face many challenges, but greater obstacles have been overcome."

Suggestions that additional research is necessary or that new treatment strategies or even preventive techniques may yet be discovered need not give a false sense of hope. Rather, these thoughts may provide comfort, even if only temporarily, and serve as a vehicle for restoring order and control to a parent's world, which has become disordered and chaotic.

Finally, it becomes the counselor's responsibility to build parental confidence. One can always find something positive to say about the way in which the parent is relating to the child, facing a crisis, or managing family routines.

Providing Immediate and Relevant Advice

Short-term aid may be required, because remediable problems often create conflict within the family. Some examples of special needs that parents may have are: managing tantrums; dealing with peer taunts; improving sibling and peer relationships; fostering independence for the child; improving bed time and eating habits; structuring leisure time for the parents; and exploring options for short-term respite care for the child.

Guiding Parents Through Transition from One Special Education Placement to Another

Dembinski and Mauser (1977) have made the following suggestions for placement counseling: Conferences including both parents can reduce the possibility of family discord and distortion of information and can increase understanding and acceptance of the child's placement. The language of the conference must eliminate professional jargon. Use of descriptive behavior levels rather than diagnostic labels is desirable. This facilitates the development of a comfortable, supportive atmosphere in which the parents are free to ask questions and raise issues of concern to them. Parents welcome reading materials or references that they can consult in order to understand the child's problem. Ideally, the school should have a library of lay-oriented materials on various aspects of the child's handicapping condition available for distribution to parents. Materials could provide definitions of terms (audiology, perception, tactile, kinesthetic) along with pamphlets listing available services. For example, the parent of the learning-disabled child would benefit from definitions of hyperactivity, information about use of medication, and materials describing the diagnostic and evaluation process.

Referral to Community Resources

Obviously the school parent counselor cannot provide a full range of services. Also, it is inappropriate to spend a great deal of time with a problem that might better be serviced by another agency. Thus, the ability to assess the need, to be knowledgeable of the special programs, financial assistance, and agencies available, and then to make the appropriate match are tasks that require serious thought and profound judgment.

Indirect Service

Interdisciplinary Communication.   Frequently, when a referral is made to an outside agency, there is a tendency to breathe a sigh of relief and say, "The job is done." However, it is often necessary to monitor progress. For instance, when a physician prescribes medication for a child, it is advisable that someone serve as liaison between the school, the home, and the physician. It is helpful initially, so that the teacher and parent are alerted to anticipated behavior changes and possible side effects, and then afterward so that they can report cognitive and behavioral changes to the physician.

Consultation and Training with School Staff Members.   Counseling services here may be useful for alleviating conflicts that may arise between the home and school. For example, when parent fatigue and sadness are misinterpreted by school staff members as lack of concern and parental indifference, it is useful to acquaint staff members with the physical and emotional demands of having a handicapped child (Harris and Fong,

1985). Also, it is important to alert school administrators that some parents of handicapped children may be restricted in movement and drained financially because of time and energy spent with doctors and at hospitals. Providing free transportation and baby sitting services may be required to get the parent to school conferences and meetings (Pfeiffer and Tittler, 1983). Finally, when planning behavior management programs, it is usually wise to urge staff members to involve the parents and to encourage them to provide reinforcement at home for behavior and academic improvements acquired in school (Blumberg, 1986).

IMPLICATIONS FOR IEP DEVELOPMENT

Current literature concerning the status of the interdisciplinary team, the IEP process, and the parent role suggests that parents continue to be relatively uninvolved in the decision-making process (Clement, Zartler, and Mulick, 1983). In fact, an observational study of the IEP process as it was conducted in three school districts in North Carolina demonstrated that parents had little understanding of the complexity of all the issues involved in ensuring that their children were appropriately serviced. It was noted in addition that these parents made no requests for related services even when such requests would have been appropriate (Goldstein, Strickland, Turnbull, and Curry, 1980). Yet the federal government's intent with Public Law 94-142 was to limit the influence of any given professional within a school district and to encourage parents to participate in their children's programming (Kaiser and Woodman, 1985).

Pfeiffer (1980) has suggested that a school team member be appointed to serve as a liaison between the school and the family to confer prior to meetings. This individual would explain legal procedures and follow the family throughout the entire process. Pfeiffer (1980) believes that this could reduce duplication of effort and mixed messages, and even suggested that a "best match" be made between the parent and team member in order to guide the selection of the most appropriate parent advocate for each family.

To meet the legal requirements, the need for parent counseling and training not only must be determined by the interdisciplinary team but must as well be documented in the IEP. The law also specifies that the intensity of the service be recorded and that there be no undue delay in providing related services to the child.

In terms of assessing the need for services to parents, Pfeiffer (1980) has listed some factors relevant to how the child actually functions within the family: information regarding recent or current life stresses, feelings of competency, belief system, child-rearing practices, family expectations for the child, problem-solving style, quality of communication, interdependence, and prominent concerns and fears.

ISSUES, CONCERNS, AND RECOMMENDATIONS

It would be easy to assume that parent counseling and training are common practices among professionals who work with handicapped children, but unfortunately this is not the case. The current situation has been described as more a promise than a fact and as a need that continues to receive little more than "lip service." Reasons often cited are poorly funded programs, heavy caseloads, not enough trained professional staff members, and the fact that working mothers are rarely available during school hours (McDowell, 1976).

Unfortunately, there are additional concerns including the practicality of techniques for changing behaviors, such as behavior management strategies. Those who use and teach behavior management know the challenges well. For example, few people are thoroughly trained in behavioral principles, which are often more complex than they seem, and consequently give a false impression that such principles are simple. It is not unusual for some practitioners to overlook the fact that for the child who suffers from clinical depression, behavior strategies alone are not usually effective (Burns, 1980). Finally, parents of handicapped children often do not have the physical and emotional energy to follow through with such programs.

Another area of concern is the ability of counselors to understand the feelings and problems of parents of handicapped children. Parent counseling literature raises doubts that much understanding exists (Kramer, 1985; Luterman, 1979; Murray, 1985). Recently, Welch (1981), a professor of special education who prided herself on her glib lectures to students about the best means of serving parents, became the parent of a child with a serious disability. She described her experience in terms of the shocking and inappropriate response rendered by her professional colleagues and friends. What surprised her most was the realization that few professionals acknowledge "gut level" feelings about exceptionalities.

Notwithstanding these issues, steps can be taken to help bridge the counseling gap between the promises of the law and daily realities. They include: (1) special training and courses at the college and university level with a focus on parent training and counseling for all those who plan to work with handicapped children; (2) proper documentation of the need for parent counseling training, regardless of staff availability, and starting at the IEP level; and (3) extensive research to develop new methods for mass dissemination of knowledge and techniques relating to parent counseling and training.

Those who work with parents of handicapped children may benefit from reading first-person experiences written in the form of books and articles that describe the responsibilities and problems of caring for a handicapped child. Such measures could foster better understanding of the needs of parents.

REFERENCES

Becker, W. C. (1971). *Parents are teachers.* Champaign, IL: Research Press.

Blumberg, T. L. (1985). Parents of handicapped children: Five preconceived myths. *Communique, 14,* 4.

Blumberg, T. L. (1986). Transforming low achieving and disruptive adolescents into model students. *The School Counselor, 34*(1) 67–72.

Burns, D. D. (1980). *Feeling good: The new mood therapy.* New York: William Morrow.

Clement, D. B., Zartler, A. S., & Mulick, J. A. (1983). Ethical considerations for school psychologists in planning for special needs children. *School Psychology Review, 12,* 452–456.

Croake, J. W., & Glover, K. E. (1977). A history and evaluation of parent education. *The Family Coordinator, 26,* 151–158.

Dembinski, R. J., & Mauser, A. J. (1977). What parents of the learning disabled want from professionals. *Journal of Learning Disabilities, 10,* 578–584.

Education of the Handicapped Regulations. (1985). 34 Code of Federal Regulations Part 300, Supplement 138.

Goldstein, S., Strickland, B., Turnbull, A. P., & Curry, L. (1980). An observational analysis of the IEP conference. *Exceptional Children, 46*(4), 278–285.

Harris, S. L., & Fong, P. L. (1985). Developmental disabilities: The family and the school. *School Psychology Review, 14,* 162–165.

Kaiser, S. M., & Woodman, R. W. (1985). Multidisciplinary teams and group decision making techniques: Possible solutions to decision making problems. *School Psychology Review, 14,* 457–470.

Kramer, J. J. (1985). Best practices in parent training. In A. Thomas & J. Grimes (Eds.), *Best practices in school psychology* (pp. 263–273). Kent, OH: The National Association of School Psychologists.

Luterman, D. M. (1979). Counseling parents of the deaf child. In E. L. Meyen (Ed.), *Basic readings in the study of exceptional children and youth* (pp. 422–429). Denver: Love Publishing Co.

McDowell, R. L. (1976). Parent counseling: The state of the art. *Journal of Learning Disabilities, 9,* 614–619.

Murray, J. N. (1985). Best practices in working with families of handicapped children. In A. Thomas & J. Grimes (Eds.), *Best practices in school psychology* (pp. 321–330). Kent, OH: The National Association of School Psychologists.

O'dell, S. (1974). Training parents in behavior modification: A review. *Psychological Bulletin, 81,* 418–433.

Patterson, G. R. (1971). *Families.* Champaign, IL: Research Press.

Pfeiffer, S. I. (1980). The school based interprofessional team: Recurring problems and some possible solutions. *Journal of School Psychology, 18,* 388–394.

Pfeiffer, S. I., & Tittler, B. I. (1983). Utilizing the multidisciplinary team to facilitate a school-family systems orientation. *School Psychology Review, 12,* 168–173.

Shapero, S., & Forbes, C. R. (1981). A review of involvement programs for parents of learning disabled children. *Journal of Learning Disabilities, 14,* 499–504.

Suran, B. G., & Rizzo, J. V. (1979). *Special children: An integrative approach.* Glenview, IL: Scott, Foresman.

Van Osdol, W. R., & Shane, D. G. (1982). *An introduction to exceptional children.* Dubuque, IA: Wm. C. Brown.

Welch, O. (1981). I know how it feels: a plea for compassionate counseling. *The Exceptional Parent, 11,* 25–26.

Chapter 9

Physical Therapy

Samuel H. Esterson

Physical therapy is primarily concerned with preventing or minimizing disability, relieving pain, improving sensorimotor function, and assisting an individual to his or her greatest physical potential following injury, disease, loss of a body part, or congenital disability. As a related service under Public Law 94-142, physical therapy assists a handicapped child to achieve maximum function in the classroom by training and working with the child in positioning, balance, range of motion (ROM), activities of daily living (ADL) skills, transfer skills, improvement of strength, speed, and accuracy of gross and fine motor skills, and improvement of motor function as an adjunct to cognitive processing received in the classroom.

DEFINITION OF PHYSICAL THERAPY

Public Law 94-142 makes a brief reference to physical therapy as "services provided by a qualified physical therapist" (Education of the Handicapped Regulations, 1985).

The physical therapist is a highly trained health professional who has completed a minimum of a four-year college program, consisting of two years preparatory liberal arts and science coursework followed by two years of basic sciences and clinical and practical physical therapy education. Physical therapy educational programs are affiliated with colleges, universities, and medical schools and are accredited by the American Physical Therapy

Association (APTA). Upon successful completion of such a program, including several months of diversified, supervised clinical education and internships in hospital settings, rehabilitation centers, schools, or private practices, an individual is eligible to take the state licensure examination. Although state standards for certification and licensure vary, each state grants a license to practice physical therapy after the individual has passed the examination.

Since the implementation of Public Law 94-142, many physical therapists have continued their graduate programs in education in specialty areas such as developmental disabilities, motor learning, and pediatric physical therapy. In addition, extended continuing education courses, such as the eight-week Neurodevelopmental Treatment (NDT) Approach to Cerebral Palsy course, have been sought by physical therapists to further their understanding and expertise in treating developmental disabilities and the neurologically impaired child.

Referrals

Referral for physical therapy is usually made by a physician. The physician submits the necessary background history of the child and appropriate medical information. This saves the physical therapist the added need for obtaining the information. Periodic therapeutic progress reports from the physical therapist to the physician are helpful in aiding the physician in the total care and treatment of the child.

Recently, several states have enacted legislation allowing a physical therapist to evaluate and treat without physician referral. In those states, the physical therapists may accept referrals from school nurses, teachers, speech-language pathologists, occupational therapists, and parents.

Candidates for Physical Therapy

Characteristics of children most frequently referred for physical therapy include:

Poor or absent sitting posture or head control
Favoring one side of the body over the other (asymmetry)
Progressive weakness and muscle wasting (atrophy)
Musculoskeletal or neuromuscular disability
Delayed developmental milestone achievement
Poor motor control, disturbed balance, and perceptual dysfunction
Absence of a limb or traumatic amputation
Curvature of the spine (scoliosis)
Wheelchair bound
Obvious gait deviation
Severe respiratory disease, such as asthma and cystic fibrosis

On the basis of these characteristics, the physical therapist commonly sees children with cerebral palsy, spina bifida, muscular dystrophy, club foot, traumatic head injury, spinal cord injury, juvenile rheumatoid arthritis, and minimal brain dysfunction.

RELATIONSHIP TO SPECIAL EDUCATION

In a large majority of school systems, physical therapy was provided to the orthopedically handicapped population long before the passage of Public Law 94-142. Since the law's enactment, the educational-therapeutic team approach to education has expanded.

Prior to Public Law 94-142, physical therapy was usually provided in isolation from the general educational program, with minimal or no contact and cooperation between the physical therapist and the special or regular education teacher. This poor cooperative effort and communication was probably due in part to the therapists' training and philosophy of working within a purely medical model and the classroom teachers' experience solely in the educational or cognitive model. Although many teachers' professional training and expertise encompass gross, fine, and perceptual motor skills, functional and self-help skills, reading, writing, communication, and vocational skill achievement, the physical therapist is trained in clinical, neurological background with expertise in identifying, evaluating, and treating muscle tone problems, orthopedic abnormalities, and reflex facilitation and inhibition techniques (Noie, 1983).

The need for better cooperation between the teacher and the physical therapist may be illustrated by an example. In a neurologically impaired child, such as one with cerebral palsy, achievement of normal gross motor skills is often infinitely complicated and greatly delayed by the presence of primitive reflex postures. These postures, which are influenced by the child's head or body in space, may cause extraneous or involuntary movements and loss of coordination, balance control, or synchrony, which neurologically intact children do not experience (Johnson and Magrab, 1976). In view of the fact that the concept of the least restrictive environment has resulted in the placement of some severely physically handicapped children in regular classrooms, the regular teacher is often not familiar with therapeutic interventions and goals, and may be facilitating and reinforcing abnormal postures and behaviors that the physical therapist is working to inhibit.

Within the guidelines of Public Law 94-142, the physical therapist is called upon to identify, evaluate, formulate an intervention plan for, and treat handicapped children to enable them to benefit from special education. The physical therapist should be familiar with the context of the law and provide services within the scope of the law's intent. The physical therapist's role includes open communication and tactful consultation with educators about evaluation findings, appropriate team intervention, and skill achievement that the child requires to function optimally within the learning environment.

Thus, physical therapy in the special education environment is directed toward the development and enhancement of the handicapped child's physical potential for maximal independence and function in all educational activities.

ELIGIBILITY FOR RELATED SERVICE PROVISION

The determination of a child's need for physical therapy is assessed by the physical therapist. The evaluation includes a history from the care-giver; the physical therapist's observation of the child's posture, strength, and movement abilities, including ambulation skills and balance; passive movement of the child's head, trunk, and limbs; palpation of the involved body segments; and assessment of the respiratory system. Close examination of the "quality" of movement and muscle tone is emphasized.

Normal posture, movement, and coordinated control of the body are possible only with the full cooperation and synchronization of the child's neurological, skeletal, and soft tissue systems.

The physical therapy evaluation may also include screening procedures, which consist of examining large numbers of children and identifying those demonstrating physical problems (Schifani, Anderson, and Odle, 1980).

More often, the physical therapist conducts an individualized and detailed evaluation of a child who displays or has a past medical history of a physical disability or handicapping condition. With skills and evaluative tools unique to physical therapy, the therapist may include the following areas in his evaluation:

Joint range of motion. The child's limbs are moved by the therapist through their full capability and the range available at each joint is measured and recorded.

Sensory and motor development. The child's ability to move on his or her own is observed and recorded. Specific attention is directed to coordination, freedom and production of movement, control of movement, balance, position of body and other limbs when moving one extremity, and tactile prehension abilities. Not only is the quantity of movement assessed, but, more important, the quality of the child's movement is closely examined.

Perceptual motor development. The child's awareness of his or her body parts and objects in space and abilities to function in his or her spatial environment are examined and recorded. Balance in all positions and coordination are also observed.

Postural reflex maturation. Primarily for the neurologically damaged child, this area addresses the child's nervous system's level of functioning, as a whole. Testing entails seeking the presence or absence of primitive and neonatal withdrawal and postural reflexes, which if present in a school-age child can severely impair or delay a child's ability to achieve normal developmental milestones, such as head control, rolling, sitting, and walking.

Oral motor skills. The child's feeding and speech abilities are examined and recorded. A close inspection is made of the child's lip closure, tongue movement, swallowing capabilities, sound production, and level of speech.

Activities of daily living (ADL) skills. The functional movement tasks associated with planning and executing grooming, hygiene, dressing, transferring, toileting, locomotion, propulsion, ambulation, and school demands are observed, analyzed, and recorded. Any task required of a child to function during a normal day is considered ADL.

Postural and gait deviations. The physical therapist closely examines the child's gait characteristics—cadence, stride, posture, endurance, and floor contact—and records the gait deviations from the norm. Structural deviations, such as scoliosis, lateral spinal curvature, leg length discrepancies, and limb anomalies are noted.

Adaptive equipment and assistive devices. The need for canes, crutches, walkers, wheelchairs, bolsters, rolls, prone boards, individualized seating construction, and other aids to maximize the child's independence in ADL, mobility, and educational performance is assessed and recorded.

Prosthetic and orthotic needs. Splint, brace, and artificial limb requirements are measured for, noted, and fitted by the physical therapist.

Respiratory system. Auscultation (listening to the air flow in the child's lungs with a stethoscope) and percussion (manual tapping of the child's lung fields to identify poor or problematic air flow regions) are performed and abnormalities are noted.

By interpreting the results of these specialized evaluations, the physical therapist determines the child's medical, physical, and functional abilities and formulates an individualized, tailored therapeutic program to facilitate optimum ability and inhibit further disability in the classroom.

OPTIONS IN SERVICE DELIVERY MODELS

The decision concerning which method of delivery of service to employ is made by an IEP committee with input from the physical therapist. The physical therapist is an integral and contributing member of the IEP committee.

Physical therapy services may be provided in the following different formats: (1) a direct, hands-on treatment session by the physical therapist;

(2) treatment by a teacher, aide, or physical therapist assistant under the supervision of a physical therapist; and (3) the physical therapist serving as a consultant to the teacher or other members of the educational and therapeutic team.

Choosing a Delivery Option

Two major factors are to be considered when determining the delivery of service options: the child's level or extent of disability and the natural progression or expected course of the diagnosis.

A child with a nonprogressive condition such as spina bifida, a condition whose progression remains static and whose disability is unchanging, would benefit from physical therapy geared toward maintaining strength and flexibility and enhancing balance reactions, mobility, activities of daily living skills and endurance. Without this physical therapy intervention, the diagnosis of spina bifida, in this case, remains unchanged; however, functional abilities, translated as *independence,* may decrease (Kalish & Presseller, 1980). A program of strengthening the non-involved muscle groups, ROM, and possibly supported standing may be prescribed by the physical therapist and implemented by the teacher or aide. Appropriate precautions and proper technique must be carefully explained to the provider of services. The physical therapist should closely monitor and reevaluate the child at established intervals and adjust the child's program as necessary.

Conversely, a child with Duchenne muscular dystrophy (a progressive, fatal neuromuscular disease) may require direct hands-on physical therapy services during periods of rapid physical regression, with frequent therapist reevaluation and program adjustment. The child's disease progression often changes, as does his or her level of disability and *dependence.*

A simpler description of the factors involved in choosing delivery of service options may be illustrated by dividing the movement and functional disability levels of the children into mild, moderate, and severe handicapping conditions. Those with mild disability may require only treatment by ancillary personnel with occasional physical therapist reevaluation and consultation; those with moderate impairment may require hands-on treatment by the physical therapist and follow-through by ancillary personnel; and the child with severe impairment may require one-on-one services rendered by the physical therapist.

Frequency and Duration of Service

Frequency of therapeutic intervention may vary from hands-on daily treatment to weekly or semimonthly. As a child receives less frequent physical therapy, the physical therapist may recommend that the IEP committee assign ancillary personnel, including the teacher, to provide care under the physical therapist's guidance with appropriate periodic supervision and reassessment. A child may begin by receiving physical therapy five days a week and later require service only twice weekly, after an intensive initial course of treatment. Depending upon the child's level of disability and the disease course, the frequency of physical therapy is determined.

The duration of physical therapy rendered to a child may range from several weeks to an entire school year. For example, a multiply-handicapped, partially ambulatory child with a non-progressive disease who is beginning to walk with an assistive device (e.g., cane, crutch, or walker) may require treatment to facilitate appropriate balance reactions, reciprocal gait pattern, range of motion, and endurance training. A learning-disabled child whose disability is not changing but whose level of function is not age appropriate may benefit from a semester of intensive physical therapy. An emotionally disturbed child in a regular school who fractured a leg in a car accident and requires physical therapy to assist in crutch ambulation training and endurance activities may need physical therapy for only several weeks until he or she becomes an independent, safe ambulator.

Location of Service Delivery

Physical therapy services may be provided in a state-of-the-art-equipped therapy suite within the school, in other areas of the school, such as the classroom, gymnasium, hallways, and stairways (especially for gait training), or at home. For functional training, the aim is to attempt to work in a setting as close to reality as possible. For example, if a child has difficulty in ascending the stairs to get to his class, the physical therapist should devote time to training the child on the steps in question. If a child demonstrates difficulty in toilet transfers, therapy sessions should take place in the lavatory.

Service Delivery by Other Personnel

The role of the physical therapist as a consultant and supervisor of assistants, teachers, and classroom aides in performing routine exercise regimens, positioning, and activities of daily living training is strongly encouraged. It is certainly not realistic to believe that every physically handicapped student in a regular, mainstreamed, or special educational environment will receive daily, hands-on, intensive physical therapy. Physical therapy manpower remains in great demand, and the number of children in need of therapeutic intervention is constantly increasing. No immediate solution to this imbalance of supply and demand is within reach. At present, the most efficient solution is for the physical therapist to delegate routine management of maintenance skills and to treat only those students requiring direct services.

IMPLICATIONS FOR IEP DEVELOPMENT

The variables of frequency and duration of physical therapy services pre-scribed for a child should be recorded on the child's individualized educa-tion program (IEP). They should be listed as annual goals or short- or long-term objectives. These variables must be agreed upon by the members of the IEP committee as well as by the parents. When there is disagreement and a mutually satisfactory solution is not agreed upon, a request for an impartial due process hearing may be made by either party.

The physical therapist, in his or her screening process, should establish criteria for evaluation of the child's extent of disability, based on chronolog-ical age, current physical therapy services received, and, most important, potential for improvement or, at least, maintenance of present functional level, in order to determine therapeutic priorities (American Physical Ther-apy Association, 1980). All of these factors influence the frequency and duration of treatment prescribed.

The physical therapist should be involved in the development of the child's IEP and also should make recommendations to improve and enhance the child's ability to fully participate and actively engage in all educational activities.

ISSUES, CONCERNS, AND RECOMMENDATIONS

As more severely impaired and multihandicapped children enter public and private classrooms, the extent of the physical therapist's training and ability to evaluate, treat, consult and provide adequate service to handicapped children comes into question. Several hypothetical questions come to light: Disease processes such as those types of cancer that occur in children are now being medically managed to the extent that affected children are living longer and are able to return to the classroom. Is the physical therapist prepared and equipped to address the multitude of precautions and special-ized treatment involved in providing service to this population? How does a physical therapist unfamiliar with sign language communicate with a physi-cally handicapped child with profound deafness who communicates in sign? Do all physical therapy programs provide adequate entry-level pediatric training to enable their graduates to be employed by a school system under educational, nontherapist supervision? Are physical therapists informed of the special education teacher's role within the school system? Should there be a special licensing or registry examination that, upon successful comple-tion, allows a physical therapist to work in the school system? Should all school system–based physical therapists be required to complete the Neuro-developmental Treatment Approach to Cerebral Palsy course?

Equipment availability is becoming a major concern for school-based therapists. Modern and sophisticated exercise equipment developed for the comprehensive treatment of the physically handicapped is often prohibitive. Therapeutic modalities, such as pools, are often not available. Without appropriate and specialized equipment, some physical therapy services cannot be properly provided.

Because many school districts employ an insufficient number of physical therapists to provide a full range of services to handicapped children, one way to alleviate the therapist shortage or the school system's inability to recruit adequate staffing is to consider contracting with private physical therapists or private practices able to supply trained and experienced personnel, supervision, management, and continuing education. Another option may be for a school system to develop an arrangement with a local hospital or clinic to provide physical therapy, equipment, and consultation.

In this chapter, several references were made to therapist-educator cooperation and consultation. It is truly unfortunate that most physical therapy education curricula are devoid of, or offer minimal exposure to, school system management, documentation of IEP goals, and the importance of the therapist-teacher relationship. As the physical therapy field of expertise and the population receiving therapeutic intervention grow, the physical therapy education curricula must expand to include such topics in their coursework.

REFERENCES

American Physical Therapy Association. (1980). Physical therapy practice in educational environments: Policies, guidelines, and background information. (Publication #P-19). Fairfax, VA: American Physical Therapy Association.

Education of the Handicapped Regulations. (1985). 34 Code of Federal Regulations Part 300, Supplement 138.

Johnson, R. B., & Magrab, P. R. (Eds.). (1976). *Developmental disorders, treatment and education.* Baltimore: University Park Press.

Kalish, R. A., & Presseller, S. (1980). Physical and occupational therapy. *Journal of School Health, 50*(5), 264–267.

Noie, D. R. (1983). Occupational and physical therapy as related services. *Teaching Exceptional Children, 15*(2), 105–107.

Schifani, J. W., Anderson, R. M., & Odle, S. J. (1980). Implementing learning in the least restrictive environment. Baltimore: University Park Press.

The Council for Exceptional Children. (1977). *PL 94-142 and Section 504— Understanding what they are and are not.* Reston, VA: The Council for Exceptional Children.

Chapter **10**

Psychological Services

Lois Therres Pommer

This chapter discusses the role of the psychologist as defined under Public Law 94-142 related service provision of "psychological services." Psychological services may be provided in the classroom (consultation to teachers or observation of children in the classroom), in a small group (group testing or group psychological counseling), individually in the psychologist's office (intelligence testing or psychological counseling), and at interdisciplinary team meetings (for sharing assessment results or setting up behavior management systems).

DEFINITION OF PSYCHOLOGICAL SERVICES

The definition of the related service "psychological services" contained in Public Law 94-142 is as follows:

(i)   Administering psychological and educational tests, and other assessment procedures;

(ii)   Interpreting assessment results;

(iii)   Obtaining, integrating, and interpreting information about child behavior and conditions relating to learning;

(iv)   Consulting with other staff members in planning school programs to meet the special needs of children as indicated by psychological tests, interviews, and behavioral evaluations; and

(v)   Planning and managing a program of psychological services, including psychological counseling for children and parents. (Education of the Handicapped Regulations, 1985).

In addition to federal special education legislation, each state has an education code that describes the function of a school psychologist in that state. To some extent, each local education agency defines the role of the school psychologist in terms of its state code. Additionally, the National Association for School Psychologists suggests appropriate roles and responsibilities of a school psychologist, with individual state associations for school psychologists defining the duties even more specifically.

RELATIONSHIP TO SPECIAL EDUCATION

Under the broad rubric "related services," there is a qualifier that psychological services are provided whenever these services assist a handicapped child to benefit from special education. In accordance with Public Law 94-142, assistance includes the early identification and assessment of handicapping conditions in children.

ELIGIBILITY FOR RELATED SERVICE PROVISION

At each individualized education program (IEP) committee meeting, the eligibility or potential need for related services, including psychological services, should be discussed. The determination that a handicapped child needs psychological services should be made by the team after considering the input of the psychologist. The following situations are examples of the need for psychological services:

1. The parents of a three-year-old girl who appears to be "slow" request a psychological evaluation to determine whether or not their daughter is mentally retarded. That child is entitled to such an evaluation.
2. A boy in a special education class for multihandicapped children becomes withdrawn, refusing to talk or make eye contact. His teachers suspect that he is suicidal. Moreover, his grades drop from As to Ds. That boy is entitled to psychological services to determine his emotional status and possible need for counseling.
3. A nine-year-old in a regular fourth grade class is reading at a preprimer level, and his mother or teacher suspects that he has a learning disability. He is entitled to psychological services to determine whether or not he is handicapped.

OPTIONS IN SERVICE DELIVERY MODELS

The provision and delivery of the various psychological services are described individually. In all cases, the services are provided by a psychologist, psychometrist, or psychology intern working under the supervision of a psychologist or psychometrist, depending upon state standards.

Administering Psychological and Educational Tests and Other Assessment Procedures

In Public Law 94-142, Regulation 300.532, Evaluation Procedures, the minimum requirements for evaluations are described as follows:

(a) Tests and other evaluation materials:
   (1) Are provided and administered in the child's native language or other mode of communication, unless it is clearly not feasible to do so;
   (2) Have been validated for the specific purpose for which they are used; and
   (3) Are administered by trained personnel in conformance with the instructions provided by their producer;
(b) Tests and other evaluation materials include those tailored to assess specific areas of educational need and not merely those which are designed to provide a single general intelligence quotient;
(c) Tests are selected and administered so as best to ensure that when a test is administered to a child with impaired sensory, manual, or speaking skills, the test results accurately reflect the child's aptitude or achievement level or whatever other factors the test purports to measure, rather than reflecting the child's impaired sensory, manual, or speaking skills (except where those skills are the factors which the test purports to measure);
(d) No single procedure is used as the sole criterion for determining an appropriate educational program for a child; and
(e) The evaluation is made by a multidisciplinary team or group of persons, including at least one teacher or other specialist with knowledge in the area of suspected disability;
(f) The child is assessed in all areas related to the suspected disability, including, where appropriate, health, vision, hearing, social and emotional status, general intelligence, academic performance, communicative status, and motor abilities.

Often, the selection of appropriate psychological and educational tests is problematic at best. Issues surrounding the possible racial and cultural bias of IQ tests have plagued psychologists, educators, parents, and others, as indicated by numerous law suits (*Larry P. v. Riles,* 1979; *Parents in Action v. Hannon,* 1980). Moreover, methodological problems abound. Few tests have been normed on specialized (that is, handicapped) populations. Yet Regulation 300.532 of Public Law 94-142 states that tests must be validated for the specific purpose for which they are used. Some handicapped children can be given standardized tests in the prescribed manner but others cannot. For some handicapped children, the test results may reflect their disability rather than their ability. At times, most psychologists have modified tests for use with handicapped children. However, scores obtained under nonstandard conditions produce uncorroborated generalizations with questionable reliability and validity. Nevertheless, adaptations of standardized testing instruments or procedures are necessary in order to test some handicapped children at all. For all handicapping conditions, a modification frequently employed is an extension of time limits. Other adaptations commonly made are listed here according to handicapping condition.

Visually Impaired.   Psychologists frequently supply large-print answer sheets, braille stimuli, tape-recorded stimuli, or oral reading by the examiner with oral responses from the visually impaired test taker.

Deaf and Hard-of-Hearing.   Depending upon the extent of the hearing impairment, psychologists may need to use sign language or use an interpreter who signs. Often, there is a reduced use of language by the examiner and a reduced emphasis on the verbal expression of the child. An increased emphasis is placed on visual and spatial abilities (that is, anything involving the interpretation of space).

Deaf-Blind.   This population generally is tested with concrete objects and a hand-over-hand approach.

Speech-Impaired.   For some speech-impaired children, such as those who stutter and some of those with impaired articulation, no adaptations may be needed. If the child's impairment is such that speech is unintelligible, a teacher who is more accustomed to the child's speech may act as a "translator." Psychologists may ask some speech-impaired children to write their responses or may choose tests for them with formats permitting a pointing or multiple-choice response.

Specific Learning-Disabled.   The most common testing modification used with learning-disabled children is out-of-level testing (that is, administering a test designed for a specific grade level to a child at another grade level). This creates methodological problems only when the test does not have out-of-level norms (scoring information provided for children outside of the intended grade level of the test). For example, if an eighth-grade child is reading at the third-grade level, the examiner may choose to give him or her a third-grade reading test. If norms are provided for children of various ages and grade placements, there is no problem. However, if the test was normed only on third-grade children, the examiner will not be able to obtain a defensible, methodologically appropriate score for the eighth-grade child.

Mentally Retarded.   As noted with the handicapping condition of specific learning disability, the psychologist may have to do out-of-level testing with the mentally retarded. The psychologist also may need to repeat or reword instructions or give concrete examples to ensure understanding.

Orthopedically Impaired.   Depending upon the nature of the orthopedic impairment(s), the child may not be able to do fine motor tasks. In these cases, the psychologist may omit certain tasks and accept verbal responses in place of written ones. The psychologist may manipulate the test materials according to the child's verbal instructions or head movements. With some severely orthopedically impaired children, the psychologist may use a multiple-choice format by which the child's eye movements indicate his or her responses. Recent developments with computers and adaptive equipment may give rise to additional modifications for this population.

Other Health-Impaired.   Generally, no special adaptations or modifications are needed for this population. Occasionally, however, the psychologist may need to extend time limits or break the testing session down into several short sessions.

Seriously Emotionally Disturbed.   More often than not, a wide range of modifications must be employed for testing seriously emotionally disturbed children. With children who refuse to speak, only nonverbal testing may be done. With overactive, acting-out children, frequent breaks may need to be taken, and testing may need to be given over several days. Special testing circumstances used to gain the cooperation of the seriously emotionally disturbed child may border on the bizarre. One psychologist allowed an emotionally disturbed adolescent to put on earphones and pretend someone from outer space was asking the questions. Another boy would cooperate only as long as he could sing a nursery rhyme between questions.

Multihandicapped.   Any of the adaptations listed for other handicapped children may apply, depending upon the nature of the multiple handicaps.

Conclusion

In general, there is a paucity of research regarding the effects of deviating from standardized test administration procedures. In order to be technically valid, methodological studies would need to be performed for each modification. The need for test research and development for the handicapped has not been addressed adequately by test publishers. In fact, test publishers generally have ignored the issue, perhaps owing to the relatively small numbers of individuals involved and the high cost of doing such studies. This fact leads to a reliance on the creativity and clinical sensitivity of the psychologist, attributes not addressed in special education legislation.

Interpreting Assessment Results

Because the results of assessment play such a pivotal role in determining whether a handicapped child is placed in a partial or full mainstreaming situation, self-contained special education class, segregated special education day school, or residential facility, as well as whether a child receives additional psychological services as a related service, the proper interpretation of assessment results is a key role of the psychologist. This interpretation is often made more difficult for the psychologist by the lack of norms for

specialized populations and the other methodological flaws addressed earlier. Furthermore, accurate interpretation requires the integration of quanti-
tative information (test scores) with qualitative information (observations
and general impressions).

Obtaining, Integrating, and Interpreting Information About Child Behavior

The psychologist obtains information on a child's behavior and learning in
many ways: observing the child in the classroom, observing the child during free periods, interviewing the child, interviewing the child's teacher,
interviewing the child's parent(s), reviewing the child's cumulative school
records, and testing the child, including projective testing (use of a drawing,
completion of a sentence, or interpretation of a picture). This information,
then, is integrated into an interpretation of the total child's behavior and
learning. In this instance, the psychologist utilizes the wealth of his or her
many years of education in order to provide information and understanding
of one individual child. This information is shared at IEP meetings, in written reports, and in consultations with parents and teachers.

Consulting With Other Staff Members in Planning School Programs

This consultation function of the psychologist occurs most frequently at IEP
meetings. Not only is the information from psychological tests, interviews,
and behavioral evaluations used for placement purposes; it is also a critical
component for curricula planning or educational programming. The psychologist shares with other staff members and the child's parent(s) information regarding the child's general intellectual functioning, modality
strengths and weaknesses, social-emotional status, and behavioral status.
These data are used in conjunction with data from other school personnel
and the child's parent(s), thus providing a system of checks and balances.

Planning and Managing a Program of Psychological Services

A provision under Public Law 94-142 mandates that each local education
agency (LEA) must have a plan for the provision and management of psychological services to students in its jurisdiction. Moreover, the provision includes
the need to have a program of psychological counseling for children and their
parents. Psychological counseling may occur in a group or one-to-one situation. It is separate from the specific counseling provided under other related
services. For example, Regulation 300.13 of Public Law 94-142 states that the
related service of audiology includes counseling and guidance of pupils, parents, and teachers regarding hearing loss. It further indicates that the related

service of social work includes group and individual counseling with the child and family. Public Law 94-142 also notes that the related service of speech pathology involves "counseling and guidance of parents, children and teachers regarding speech and language disorders." More broadly, there is a related service of counseling services, which may be provided by qualified social workers, psychologists, guidance counselors, or other qualified personnel, and a related service of parent counseling and training, which requires assisting parents in understanding the special needs of their child and providing parents with information about child development.

IMPLICATIONS FOR IEP DEVELOPMENT

The individualized education program known as IEP is a written statement, containing levels of educational performance, annual goals, the specific special education and related services to be provided to the child, dates for initiation and duration of services, and criteria and procedures for determining the acquisition of instructional objectives. It is used to monitor the child's educational progress and the effectiveness of his or her educational program. Briefly stated, the purpose of the IEP is to promote accountability.

If the IEP committee determines that a child is eligible for psychological services, the specific components and extent of such services are delineated on the IEP. Psychological services need to be included in the IEP only when they differ from services provided to nonhandicapped students. Some examples will illustrate this point:

1. A school system administers the Slosson Intelligence Test to all children as part of the standardized group testing process. That psychological testing service would not need to be recorded on the IEP because it is not unique to the handicapped child's special education or related service needs.
2. A mentally retarded child will be transferring from an elementary school to a middle school at the start of the following school year. The IEP development team determines that psychological tests should be administered to the child in order to update ability and functional levels. The plan for that child's psychological testing should be recorded on the IEP.

ISSUES, CONCERNS, AND RECOMMENDATIONS

For many years, a critical issue for psychologists has been the overidentification of minorities as handicapped. The central issue in the federal courts case of *Larry P. v. Riles* (1979) was the allegation that general aptitude tests were racially and culturally biased against blacks, who were subsequently misclassified as mentally retarded. To safeguard against potential errors in identification, psychologists must use adaptive behavior measures in addition to standardized intelligence measures. The very use of standardized instruments implies some fairness among all populations included in the norm sample. As noted by Anastasi (1982), "when social stereotypes and prejudice may distort interpersonal evaluations, tests provide a safeguard against favoritism and arbitrary or capricious decisions."

The author believes there is a strong need for additional test development and research for handicapped populations. Tests need to be standardized on specific handicapped populations; test publishers need to include appropriate percentages of various handicapped children in the norming sample; and existing tests need to be re-normed with modifications for the handicapped. Without these provisions, the reliability and validity of standardized test instruments are uncertain at best. There is additional controversy about the poor reliability of infant intelligence tests, which is of special significance for states serving children at birth. This is a major difficulty that has not been addressed by the test developers and that warrants intense investigation.

Controversy exists over funding for children receiving services or needing services from more than one agency. The educational agency is the only agency mandated with such specific guidelines as provided in Public Law 94-142. However, some agencies share in the responsibility for a child's care, and interagency collaboration is becoming more visible. This cooperative arrangement requires agencies to delineate their roles and fiscal responsibilities.

In order to provide psychological services, the psychologist must be able to work with individual children, gaining their confidence and rapport, with groups of children, with individual adults, and with groups of adults. The psychologist needs to have much technical knowledge and an ability to integrate information from a variety of sources. Only when these conditions are present will the psychologist meet the intent of the law in providing psychological services to handicapped children.

REFERENCES

Anastasi, A. (1982). Psychological testing (5th ed.). New York: Macmillan.

Education of the Handicapped Regulations. (1985). 34 Code of Federal Regulations Part 300, Supplement 138.

Larry P. v. Riles, No. C-71-2770 RFP. Northern District, CA (1979).

Parents in Action on Special Education v. Hannon, No. 74-C-3586. Northern District, IL (1980).

Chapter 11

Recreation

Morton M. Esterson

Today, with the ever-increasing amount of available leisure time due to unemployment, advances in medical and scientific technology, improved health standards and longer life spans, the need for recreation and leisure pursuits is becoming more important. Education for the worthy use of leisure time was one of the cardinal principles espoused in 1917 by the Commission on the Reorganization of Secondary Education and continues to be a high priority.

All children, handicapped and nonhandicapped, require an educational program that includes instruction in the constructive use of leisure time and recreation. Bender, Brannan, and Verhoven (1984) note that although special education has demonstrated interest in providing a comprehensive curriculum for many handicapped children, recreation and leisure activities are generally considered a low priority in most school curriculums. How ironic it is that handicapped children, who have the greatest need for recreation and leisure skill training, receive the least amount of preparation and training in these areas during their school years. This is truly a sad commentary on the education of the handicapped that many children, having completed their program of study and sorely lacking in recreational skills, have so little to look forward to each day.

DEFINITION OF RECREATION

According to Public Law 94-142, recreation is a related service consisting of (1) assessment of leisure function; (2) therapeutic recreation services; (3) recreation programs in schools and community agencies; and (4) leisure education (Education of the Handicapped Regulations, 1985).

Continuing to emphasize the importance of recreation and extracurricular activities for the handicapped, Public Law 94-142 states:

(a) Each public agency shall take steps to provide nonacademic and extracurricular services and activities in such manner as is necessary to afford handicapped children an equal opportunity for participation in those services and activities.

(b) Nonacademic and extracurricular services and activities may include counseling services, athletics, transportation, health services, recreational activities, special interest groups or clubs sponsored by the public agency, referrals to agencies which provide assistance to handicapped persons, and employment of students, including both employment by the public agency and assistance in making outside employment available (Education of the Handicapped Regulations, 1985).

By enacting Public Law 94-142, the U.S. Congress affirmed the rights of handicapped children to a free appropriate public education at no cost to parents or guardians. The federal law requires that each state education agency assume the responsibility for ensuring that public agencies establish and implement the goal of providing an educational opportunity to all the handicapped children they serve. In addition, Congress encouraged all local education agencies to offer artistic and cultural activities to the handicapped.

Excerpts from the Senate Report on Public Law 94-142 highlight the importance of providing recreational types of activities as related services to handicapped children:

> The use of the arts as a teaching tool for the handicapped has long been recognized as a viable, effective way not only of teaching special skills, but also of teaching youngsters who had otherwise been unteachable. The committee envisions that programs under this bill could well include an arts component and, indeed, urges that local educational agencies include the arts in programs for the handicapped funded under this Act. Such a program could cover both appreciation of the arts by the handicapped youngsters, and the utilization of the arts as a teaching tool per se.
>
> Museum settings have often been another effective tool in the teaching of handicapped children. For example, the Brooklyn Museum has been a leader in developing exhibits utilizing the heightened tactile sensory skill of the blind. Therefore, in light of the national policy concerning the use of museums in Federally supported education programs enunciated in the Education Amendments of 1974, the committee also urges local educational agencies to include museums in programs for the handicapped funded under this Act.
>
> (Senate Report No. 94-168, 1975)

RELATIONSHIP TO SPECIAL EDUCATION

Recreation, like all related services, must be required to assist the handicapped child to benefit from special education before it becomes the responsibility of the local education agency to provide the service.

For severely and profoundly handicapped children, recreation activities are necessary for the purpose of initiating greater pride and independence and should therefore be considered an integral component of their special education programs. Heward and Orlansky (1980) report that "socialization skills, eye-hand coordination, physical development, cognitive or language development may also be increased through therapeutic recreation."

The term "therapeutic recreation" has been defined by the National Recreation and Park Association (1978) as a process that utilizes recreation services for purposeful intervention in some physical, emotional, or social behavior, in order to bring about a desired change in that behavior and to promote the growth and development of the child.

The provision of recreation as a related service affords local education agencies the opportunity to integrate handicapped children in the least restrictive environment together with their non-handicapped peers, as implied in Public Law 94-142.

As Bender and associates (1984) observe, the American Medical Association has often reported that recreation contributes to the promotion of health, the prevention of illness and further disability, the treatment of illness, and the rehabilitation of children with physical, social, emotional, and intellectual disabilities.

Recreation for the handicapped promotes and enhances growth and personal development. Bender and associates (1984) report that the implications for the use of recreational activities can be seen in studies of the detrimental effects of isolation, hospitalization, and institutionalization and of the positive effects of physical and recreational activities.

OPTIONS FOR SERVICE DELIVERY MODELS

Opportunities for recreation can be provided before, during, or after school as well as on weekends and holidays and during vacation time. Recreation may consist of formal and informal activities and individual and group activities.

Recreational skills include the ability to amuse oneself in an appropriate manner when alone and the ability to participate with others in age-appropriate recreational environments (Sailor and Gross, 1983).

Recreation is an activity that a child selects to engage in during leisure time. Recreational activities are numerous and vary from child to child. What gives one child pleasure and satisfaction may not be considered recreation for another child. It is a personal preference.

Although it is not always reasonable to expect that all handicapped children will compete competitively with their nonhandicapped peers, they can be integrated and mainstreamed with them either as active participants or as spectators.

Recreational activities range from those that require a minimum of physical ability or prowess to those that require much concentration, exercise, training, and skill.

A suggested listing of recreation and leisure games can include numerous activities from A to Z:

aerobics	nature study
bicycling	oil painting
camping	puppetry
dancing	quoits
exercising	roller-skating
fishing	scouting
gardening	tennis
hiking	underwater sports
ice skating	volleyball
jogging	wheelchair sports
karate	xylophone playing
leather working	yachting
music	zoo tripping

Organizations such as Special Olympics, The President's Committee on the Arts for the Handicapped, The Boy Scouts of America—Scouting for the Handicapped Division, and the Girl Scouts of the USA—Scouting for Handicapped Girls sponsor recreation programs for handicapped children. Generally, local bureaus and departments of recreation cooperate with local education agencies in providing recreational activities and facilities for handicapped children.

IMPLICATIONS FOR IEP DEVELOPMENT

When the related service of recreation is recommended by a child's individualized education program committee, the specific form or type of recreation and the frequency, initiation, and duration of the service should be clearly stated in the child's IEP. Short-term and long-term goals and objectives should also be recorded.

There may be cases where transportation is required in order for the child to receive the recommended recreation service. In such cases, transportation must also be recorded on the child's IEP.

If a recreational therapist, one who is professionally trained to help handicapped children structure their use of leisure time, is recommended to provide or supervise the recreation service, the name of the therapist should be recorded on the IEP.

ISSUES, CONCERNS, AND RECOMMENDATIONS

Despite current fiscal, economic, and budgetary constraints, the opportunities for recreation and leisure will continue to increase and expand. School districts will have to place greater emphasis on teaching handicapped children more productive use of leisure and preparation for related occupations.

Meyen (1982) stresses the fact that recreation and leisure education should be incorporated into the special education curriculum beginning with preschool. This is important for all children, but especially for severely handicapped children, because recreation, which is an avocational activity, may be the one activity most important in their lives.

Because of the increasingly limited vocational and career opportunities available to handicapped children, they will have more free time; therefore, the teaching of recreation and leisure skills is of paramount importance. Collaborative efforts between local education agencies and philanthropic groups can help facilitate the inclusion in school programs of recreation as a related service for handicapped children.

Community agencies and public and private facilities must join together in promoting recreation and leisure activities for handicapped children. Public libraries, for example, supply more than just books. They offer opportunities for "story time" and "film presentations" (Katzen, 1981). In addition, many libraries lend out films, tapes, records and videocassettes.

Finally, it is important to remember that parents and advocate groups can be most influential in espousing recreation as a related service for handicapped children. This resource should not be overlooked.

REFERENCES

Bender, M., Brannan, S. A., & Verhoven, P. J. (1984). *Leisure education for the handicapped: Curriculum goals, activities, and resources.* San Diego, CA: College-Hill Press.

Education of the Handicapped Regulations. (1985). 34 Code of Federal Regulations Part 300, Supplement 138.

Heward, W. L., & Orlansky, M. D. (1980). *Exceptional children: An introductory survey to special education.* Columbus, OH: Charles E. Merrill Publishing Company.

Katzen, G. (1981, April). Your professional: The recreational therapist. *The Exceptional Parent,* p. 27.

Meyen, E. L. (1982). *Exceptional children and youth: An introduction.* Denver, CO: Love Publishing Co.

National Recreation and Park Association. (1978) *The therapeutic recreation.* (p. 1).

Sailor, W., & Guess, D. (1983). *Severely handicapped students: An instructional design.* Boston: Houghton Mifflin Co.

Senate Report No. 94-168 (1975).

Chapter **12**

School Health Services

Grace Black
Thomas V. Dorsett

Three o'clock! The school bell rings! A few minutes later, scores of children pour down the steps on their way to an afternoon of playing with friends. Among them is a small girl skipping toward a waiting bus. As she passes a classmate on a bench, she gives him a friendly tap on the shoulder. Who would ever guess that these two happy children have serious health problems? Yet if this girl and this boy, and many like them, did not receive special school health services, they would not be able to attend school. But they do. The little girl's clothing hides a gastrostomy, a feeding tube, her sole source of nourishment; the boy, waiting for his daily taxi to take him home, has a healing fracture from a rare bone disease.

These services help them overcome their handicaps and help avoid the worst handicap of all, the psychological problems that arise when children are isolated from their peers.

These children, in addition to those with seizures, birth defects, muscular diseases, cystic fibrosis, and other health impairments, will require school health services.

DEFINITION OF SCHOOL HEALTH SERVICES

Public Law 94-142 defines school health services as those services provided by a qualified school nurse or other qualified person (Education of the Handicapped Regulations, 1985).

In school districts having an adequate number of school nurses, a school nurse would provide the related health services. However, if there is a shortage of nursing personnel, a school nurse may supervise provision of the required school health services by a specially trained nonmedical person.

According to the federal definition, any qualified individual may provide or supervise the provision of health services.

Because handicapped children are often more vulnerable to communicable diseases and frequently have special health needs, the services of a school nurse are essential to them (Meyen and Lehr, 1982).

RELATIONSHIP TO SPECIAL EDUCATION

Many children with handicapping conditions will require school health services in order to benefit from special education. Without such related services, these children would be unable to attend school or remain in school for a full day.

Health services may include special feedings, catheterization, suctioning, administering medications, planning for the child's safety in school (such as securing appropriately modified physical education and preparing an evacuation plan for children with limited mobility in case of fire or other disaster), and assuring that care will be given in the classroom to prevent further injury (such as arranging for frequent position changes to prevent pressure sores).

ELIGIBILITY FOR RELATED SERVICE PROVISION

All children, whether in special education or in a regular program, are eligible for school health services. However, for a child to receive school health services without which he or she cannot remain in school, the child must have been examined by a physician, who must provide a statement that these services are necessary. Once a child is placed in a setting where the services can be provided, specific physician orders for medications or treatments are required.

School nurses and trained health assistants should be available to direct the health care given to school children. Although Public Law 94-142 mandates that school health services be provided, it does not mandate or fund nursing services. Therefore, in school systems where professional staff is scarce, many health services are provided in more restrictive settings, such as in special schools, rather than in the mainstream. Consequently, children are often placed in more restrictive settings than necessitated by their health problems.

OPTIONS IN SERVICE DELIVERY MODELS

School health services may be provided in a variety of settings or modes. The most common is in a regular classroom, with either the child's being brought to the health room or health personnel's going to the classroom to provide specialized care. In general, for care of a more intimate nature such as changing the appliance on an ostomy (an artificial opening into a body cavity for excreting waste matter), the child would go or be taken to the health room. For care of a less personal nature, such as administration of medications to a roomful of children with very limited mobility, the nurse might go to the classroom.

Because some schools were constructed before the passage of current laws mandating accessibility for the handicapped, children with limited mobility or with other problems requiring a special environment will need to be assigned to a building that is barrier free to accommodate the handicapped.

Some children, such as those with severe cardiac or respiratory problems, may need a nurse on site at all times. Children with similar types of handicaps requiring frequent nursing care can be grouped in one school. Other children who are unstable physically but able to study and learn may need to have education provided in a hospital or rehabilitation center or at home. In hospitals and rehabilitation centers, nurses are available to provide health care as needed. When a child is confined to home, periodic visits from a nurse can help to ensure that he or she is progressing physically as desired. The nurse can also offer consultation to teachers who may be unfamiliar with or fearful of the child's condition or special equipment. She can also keep the physician apprised of the child's status, to assist in determining when the child is ready for a less restrictive environment. The nurse can also inform the receiving school about what services or special arrangements will be needed to maintain the child in a less restrictive environment.

Another model of delivery of service is contracting with an agency, such as a visiting nurse association, to provide skilled service on a part-time basis. Where insufficient school nursing service exists, it may be possible for the local education agency (LEA) to purchase service from a community health care provider, whose personnel will come in daily or as needed to provide a specific skilled service, such as a tube feeding, wound care, or a sterile catheterization. Although ongoing care by a nurse to whom the child is known will give better continuity of care, this is an alternate means of providing high-quality skilled service relatively inexpensively.

IMPLICATIONS FOR IEP DEVELOPMENT

Although Public Law 94-142 does not provide a standard format for the IEP, it does require that various factors be considered in developing the IEP. All plans should include medical, developmental, and neurological considerations and their impact upon the child's progress and ability to learn. The school nurse or physician should be consulted in regard to this portion of the plan. In some systems they may actually participate in writing the plan, especially if the child needs special handling in the classroom in order to remain functional; for example, a child on insulin may need to eat lunch at a particular time to avoid a reaction to his drug; another may need a modified physical education program, or rest periods if certain symptoms arise. Inclusion of this information in the IEP can prevent harm to the child and disruption of the classroom by medical emergencies.

The physician or school nurse should submit written recommendations to the IEP committee and, whenever possible, should actively participate in the placement decision to ensure that the necessary health considerations are satisfied.

ISSUES, CONCERNS, AND RECOMMENDATIONS

Igoe and associates (1980) caution that without school nursing services, school personnel including classroom teachers face serious risks if they assume responsibility for the performance of complicated health procedures that they are neither prepared nor licensed for but that are necessary if students with certain handicaps are to receive the education to which they are entitled under Public Law 94-142. Although the courts have ruled, in at least one instance, in regard to intermittent catheterization, that the procedure need not be done by a nurse, the nursing practice acts of individual states may prohibit the performance of certain procedures by nonmedical people.

Today's registered nurse (RN) is basically prepared to provide most health services needed to maintain a child in school. In order both to ensure the safety of school children and to protect school personnel from liability for inappropriate judgment, some school nurse and nursing assistant time should be provided by every local education agency for the registered nurse to be able to evaluate each handicapped child before delegating care to an assistant. If she cannot spend all her time in one school, she should be close enough to be able to go within a half hour to any school for which she has responsibility. She should be readily accessible for telephone consultation.

Some jurisdictions have utilized licensed practical nurses (LPNs) or licensed vocational nurses (LVNs) to supplement their registered nurse staff. These nurses are prepared to do procedures such as suctioning, stoma care, and tube feedings and are licensed to perform them under the supervision of a registered nurse (RN). LPNs are better qualified to perform these services than trained nursing assistants or volunteers. Use of LPNs or LVNs under RN supervision would probably meet the standards of most states' nursing practice acts. These personnel would have more training and knowledge with which to respond to an emergency than nursing assistants or trained volunteers. Because Public Law 94-142 requires that the LEA be responsible for ensuring that related services are provided by qualified personnel, administrators would be well advised to ascertain that health personnel have a sufficient ratio not only of RNs to children with special needs, but of RNs to auxiliary personnel used in providing services. LPNs or LVNs, because of their training, require less supervision for ensuring the safety of children than assistants whose preparation is less intensive.

Recently, the United States Supreme Court clarified several health issues with regard to the interpretation of Public Law 94-142 that may serve as guides to implementing the Education of All Handicapped Children Act. Future cases of disagreement will undoubtedly be resolved by the courts.

Amber Tatro, a child attending school in 1979 in a Texas school district, had spina bifida, suffered from orthopedic and speech impairments, and also had impaired function of the urinary bladder. She required clean intermittent catheterization (CIC), because she was unable to voluntarily empty her bladder, every three to four hours so as to avoid chronic kidney infection. The local school district prepared an individualized education program for Amber but did not include CIC because they considered it a medical service. The parents disagreed with the exclusion of CIC and requested a due process hearing before an Impartial Hearing Officer. The Hearing Officer ruled in favor of the parents. The Texas Commissioner of Education adopted that decision, but it was then reversed by the State Board of Education.

The Tatros immediately filed suit in the Federal District Court. The Court declared that CIC was not a related service under Public Law 94-142 because it does not serve a need arising from the effort to educate a handicapped child. The parents appealed the decision, and the Fifth Circuit Court of Appeals, in *Tatro v. State of Texas* (1980), reversed the lower court decision by ruling that CIC was a related service for Amber Tatro because it was required if she were to attend school and benefit from special education (Piele, 1982).

In analyzing its decision, the Supreme Court provided answers to two basic questions: Is CIC a supportive service required to assist a handicapped child to benefit from special education? *and* Is CIC a medical service excluded from the definition of supportive services?

The Supreme Court Justices all agreed that in the case of Amber Tatro, CIC was a supportive service. Without such aid, she could not attend school and benefit from special education. The Justices compared CIC services that permit a child to remain in school during the day with services that enable a child to reach, enter, and exit the school. They unanimously agreed on the second question as well. They differentiated between school health services and medical services, with the former provided by a school nurse or other qualified person and the latter by a licensed physician. The Supreme Court ruled that where nonmedical health services are necessary to allow a handicapped child to benefit from special education, they qualify as supportive services and are required by federal law. They added that to be eligible for supportive services, a child must be handicapped and require special education. The Court ruled, however, that if a service can appropriately be provided other than during the school day, a school district is not required to provide it.

On January 19, 1981, the Department of Education issued a notice of interpretation (34 CFR §§ 104 and 300, 46 Fed. Reg. 4912) clarifying CIC as a related service and therefore required to be provided by school districts. The notice explains that CIC is a relatively simple procedure that can be administered with minimal training by a school nurse or any responsible person, including a child who himself or herself requires catheterization. A license is not needed to perform this service.

Although CIC is not specifically mentioned in the description of related services in Public Law 94-142, the comment following the regulation states, "The list of related services is not exhaustive and may include other developmental, corrective, or supportive services if they are required to assist a handicapped child to benefit from special education" (Education of the Handicapped Regulations, 1985). The Secretary of Education has concluded that catheterization is a related service as defined in Public Law 94-142.

The AIDS Issue

Recently, many school districts have confronted an important educational decision: Can a child who has acquired immune deficiency syndrome (AIDS) be excluded from attending school? Because all children have a basic right to a free appropriate public education, is exclusion of a child from school legal?

For school districts, this issue is most complex, because it cuts across socioeconomic, racial, and geographic lines and pits the educational, medical, and legal communities against one another. Some school districts argue that no child should be excluded from school. Other school districts would exclude children with AIDS or the AIDS virus despite the fact that all experts in this disease agree that children who have AIDS or are infected with the AIDS virus cannot spread the disease by casual contact (Reed, 1986). There is no medical reason, therefore, to prohibit a child with AIDS from attending school except under very specific circumstances.

Flygare (1986) observes that unless an AIDS victim is physically unable to attend school, school officials have little choice in the matter of whether the child can be barred from school attendance. A child with AIDS in most instances cannot be excluded from attending school unless he or she exhibits disruptive behavior.

Supporting this statement are recently issued federal guidelines, which state that children with AIDS can attend school. The first set of guidelines issued at the federal level by the Centers for Disease Control (CDC) in Atlanta on August 30, 1985, report that the benefits of attending school by most AIDS infected children far outweigh the apparently nonexistent risk of transmission of the disease. They add that the decision whether a child should attend school should be based on his or her behavior, neurological development, and physical condition. If a child lacks control of his or her body secretions, has a tendency to bite people, or has oozing lesions that cannot be covered, a more restricted environment may be appropriate (New federal guidelines, 1985).

Each school district should develop a clearly written policy regarding school attendance by children who are infected with the AIDS virus that clarifies the child's rights to a free appropriate education in the least restrictive environment. The policy should also address the topics of confidentiality of children's school records as well as the right of teachers and other school employees to know the health status of the children they teach. The AIDS guidelines should be part of more general guidelines regarding hygiene for other communicable diseases.

Recommendations

We suggest that there are three basic questions regarding the provision of school health services.

What services will be provided?
Who will provide them?
How will they be funded?

Any health service that is required to keep a child in school must be provided. Recognition, therefore, must be given to the existence of more and more children with serious handicaps who have survived high-risk pregnancy, prematurity, birth defects, and life-threatening accidents; school districts countrywide must come to grips with the fact that many children are still excluded from receiving an appropriate education or are receiving inadequate school health services. Requests from parents to involve these seriously impaired children in education outside the home are being made more frequently.

Some thought also should be given to the emotional effect that severely health impaired children, who may need highly specialized equipment, have on nonhandicapped children. Although hospitalized children remember mostly the pleasant aspects of their hospital experience and associations, some do experience fear and nightmares resulting from their observation of other seriously ill or dying children. Plans must be made for skillful dealing with frightening situations in the classroom, most suitably by psychologists, school nurses, or teachers.

In order to provide school health services in a financially feasible way to the increasing numbers of special children who need them, several actions are recommended. First, all teacher education programs should include not only a basic health course but also a mandatory course on the management of common handicapping conditions in the classroom, to demystify health conditions so that teachers can address some problems on a commonsense basis (not like the teacher who refused to give orange juice to a child having an insulin reaction, because it was a treatment).

Second, every LEA should employ or arrange with the local health department (LHD) for sufficient registered nurses trained in school health to provide appropriate care or to supervise others in the provision of care to maintain children safely in school. In subdivisions that have not provided nursing care, different means can be used, such as various mixes of registered nurses and school nurse practitioners, LPNs or LVNs and nursing assistants, and private duty nurses or aides who will in school care for a child requiring one-on-one medical care.

Third, other arrangements, like teleteaching and other types of learning experience for involving children who cannot travel to school daily, should be considered.

Fourth, at some point, unless there is a drastic change in the economy, LEAs will have to legally set some priorities for care, or systems could totally exhaust their educational resources in order to provide service for special education students. Therefore, a careful distinction must be made between what are appropriate necessities and what are not in providing related services.

Fifth, as recommended by Igoe (1980), a nationwide program of continuing education for school nurses to expand and update rehabilitation knowledge and skills should be instituted, with support and direction from the American Nurses Association's Division on Nursing Practice, The American School Health Association, and the National Association of School Nurses. It would be most appropriate for continuing education courses to be co-sponsored with educational agencies who directly serve handicapped children. A benefit of a national program in rehabilitation of the handicapped is that uniform standards of quality could be assured and information would also be available to nurses from poorer or more rural areas who might not have access to some of the excellent training programs offered in individual subdivisions.

REFERENCES

Education of the Handicapped Regulations. (1985). 34 Code of Federal Regulations Part 300, Supplement 138.

Flygare, T. J. (1986). Are victims of AIDS handicapped under federal law? *Phi Delta Kappan, 67*(6), 466–467.

Igoe, J., Green, P., Heim, H., Licata, M., Macdonough, G., McHugh, B. A., Smith, L. L., & Tjornhom, B. H. (1980). School nurses working with handicapped children: A statement of the American Nurses Association. Publication #NP-60 2M. Kansas City, MO: American Nurses Association.

Meyen, E. L., & Lehr, D. H. (Eds.). (1982). *Exceptional children in today's schools: An alternative resource book.* Denver, CO: Love Publishing Co.

New federal guidelines say children with AIDS can attend school. (1985). *Phi Delta Kappan, 67*(3), 242, 244.

Piele, P. K. (1982). *Yearbook of school law.* Topeka, KS: National Organization on Legal Problems of Education, pp. 132–133.

Reed, S. (1986). AIDS in the schools: A special report. *Phi Delta Kappan, 67*(7), 494–498.

Tatro v. *State of Texas,* 625 F.2d 557 (5th Cir. 1980).

Chapter 13

Social Work Services in Schools

Stuart M. Tabb

Social workers have a longstanding history of providing services for children with special needs in public schools. The services mandated to be provided by school social workers by Public Law 94-142, The Education For All Handicapped Children Act, are consistent with the very nature of school social work services.

A recognition of the need to consider factors beyond the schools that may be affecting a child's educational performance was noted as early as 1913 by the Rochester Board of Education, the first system to employ school social workers, at that time referred to as visiting teachers. The Board stated, "This is the first step in an attempt to meet a need of which the school system has been conscious to for some time. It is an undisputed fact that in the environment of the child outside of school are found forces which will often-times thwart the school in its endeavors. . . . The appointment of a visiting teacher is an attempt on the part of the school to meet its responsibility for the whole welfare of the child . . . and to secure maximum cooperation between the home and the school" (Oppenheimer, 1925).

DEFINITION OF SOCIAL WORK SERVICES

The Education For All Handicapped Children Act of 1975 (Public Law 94-142) defines social work services in schools to include:

(i)   Preparing a social or developmental history on a handicapped child;
(ii) Group and individual counseling with the child and family;

(iii) Working with those problems in a child's living situation (home, school, and community) that affect the child's adjustment in school; and

(iv) Mobilizing school and community resources to enable the child to receive maximum benefit from his or her educational program. (Education of the Handicapped Regulations, 1985).

The National Association of Social Workers (1977) suggests additional activities and responsibilities that school social workers should consider in providing comprehensive services to handicapped children.

Qualifications of a School Social Worker

To qualify as a school social worker, an individual must complete a two-year master's degree program from an accredited school of social work. The program includes coursework in human development, social policy, community development, social work methods for individual and group counseling, and social administration. In addition, two semesters of field placement in public or private facilities are generally required. With the master's degree and two years of supervised social work experience, the individual is eligible for state department certification as a licensed certified social worker (LCSW).

RELATIONSHIP TO SPECIAL EDUCATION

Handicapped children such as those with severe emotional and social problems may require the intervention and assistance of a social worker to enable them to adjust to their school placement. In general, social work as a related service is required if there are indications that it may "assist a handicapped child to benefit from special education" (Education of the Handicapped Regulations, 1985).

ELIGIBILITY FOR RELATED SERVICE PROVISION

As stated, social work services in schools, according to Public Law 94-142, may be provided only if they are necessary to assist a handicapped child to benefit from special education. This determination should be made by a multidisciplinary team with the input of a school social worker after a determination has been made that a child is handicapped.

For a child whose attitude or behavior has an adverse or negative affect upon educational performance, school social work services would be considered a necessary related service. They would also be seen as necessary for a child who is experiencing problems outside of school, such as within his or her family, that are adversely affecting the child's educational performance.

The following services are examples of those provided by a social worker that would be considered related services:

1. Determining special needs of children and their families within or outside the school and making appropriate referrals.
2. Preparing a social or developmental history for IEP development.
3. Counseling children and their families individually or in groups.
4. Assisting parents to participate in conferences and IEP meetings.
5. Serving as a liaison between home, school, and community (e.g., interpreting school policy to the parent or guardian; providing specific family information to the school).
6. Providing in-service and staff training to school personnel relative to a child's school adjustment or special needs.
7. Providing transitional services for children going into or coming out of special education or changing programs within special education.
8. Serving as a case manager or liaison with community-based agencies to coordinate special services.

OPTIONS IN SERVICE DELIVERY MODELS

This section is not meant to be an all-inclusive listing of social work services. It presents detailed explanations of two services that social workers may consider and that are separate from their casework or counseling roles: mediation and social assessment.

Mediation

School social workers bear "extensive responsibility and public trust" for being knowledgeable about and informational resources on federal and relevant state and local laws affecting education and school social work (Anderson, 1977). They can facilitate the implementation of such legislation, because of their specialized training and as a result of their advocacy positions.

Social workers have traditionally involved themselves in assisting individuals, families, and groups to resolve conflicts of various types. Such conflicts include those between husband and wife, parent and child, teacher and child, group member and group member, and professional and professional. Disagreements often occur between parents and school personnel about special education procedures or issues. By federal law, if these disagreements are not resolved or reconciliation cannot be reached, a parent or a public education agency may initiate a hearing into the matter. Federal regulations also allow for use of mediation "as an intervening step prior to conducting a formal due process hearing" (Education of the Handicapped Regulations, 1985).

Claire Gallant (1982), a social worker who has served as a mediator and trainer and has developed procedures for such reconciliation attempts, lists the following skills and due process knowledge necessary for an effective mediator: (1) detailed knowledge of the due process procedures of Public Law 94-142 and relevant state legislation and regulations; (2) general knowledge of special education programs and related services; (3) skill in group management; (4) skill in assimilating individual case data; (5) skill in communicating special education needs of the child; (6) skill in assessment of participants; (7) skill in resolving nonadversarial disputes; and (8) skill in writing contracts or agreements (Gallant, 1982).

A mediator must have an understanding of such areas as human behavior, group dynamics, and systems theory, as well as basic knowledge of schools, special education, and pertinent laws. As Gallant (1982) remarks, "mediation is a logical and challenging expansion of basic social work skills." The mediation process is generally more cost-effective than a formal hearing and can promote cooperative parent-school relationships that are substantially less adversarial. In mediation, the parties involved make the decision as opposed to the Hearing Officer who, in effect, would impose a decision.

The Social Assessment or Social History

The administrative regulations of Public Law 94-142 explicitly state that one function of social work services in schools is preparing a social or developmental history of a handicapped child. In assessing students for special education services and placement, the legislative mandate also requires that (1) the evaluation(s) be administered by trained personnel; (2) the evaluation be made by a multidisciplinary team; (3) no single procedure be used as the sole criterion for determining an appropriate educational program; and (4) the child be assessed in all areas related to the suspected disability, including where appropriate the child's social and emotional status (Education of the Handicapped Regulations, 1985).

The Virginia State Board of Education (1972) emphasizes the fact that the sociological component is a critical part of any such diagnosis. "In evaluating the 'total' child, it is necessary that the social worker considers the family dynamics and home environmental situation influencing a child's learning and behavioral patterns. Such information is invaluable in making a comprehensive appraisal of the child's difficulty. Communication and cooperation with the family must be established and maintained in order to facilitate environmental change necessary to correct learning and/or behavioral problems" (Wilkerson, 1977).

The primary purpose of the social history is to aid in the educational placement of the child. A secondary purpose of the social history is to help "guard against the inappropriate labeling of children based on test scores and school performance alone without consideration of cultural and language differences" (Byrne, Hare, Hooper, Morse, and Sabatino, 1977).

In addition to being a "fact finder" of sorts in developing a social history, the social worker may act as a short-term counselor, providing support and information to the parent(s); as a referral agent when information gathered suggests the appropriateness of such an action; and as an advocate, informing parents of such matters as their due process rights and placement options. The process for gathering information, particularly the parent interview, should be a dynamic process and could be a valuable tool in developing a positive relationship with parent(s). It also can set a precedent for continued cooperation in the evaluation-placement process.

Generally, a social history written by a social worker would include the following components: (1) reason for referral or details regarding the presenting problem(s); (2) developmental history with attention to suspected delays or physiological impediments; (3) medical history, including frequency of illness, injuries, or hospitalizations; (4) school history; (5) family history and social data; (6) summary or evaluation synthesizing all the information; and (7) recommendations regarding special educational services and other areas of potential follow-up.

The social history can be used dynamically as both a comprehensive assessment tool and as a strategy for short-term casework intervention. In this way, the product can be utilized as a critical component, incorporating essential pieces of background information and present functioning, in formulating an educational plan in consideration of the "whole child."

IMPLICATIONS FOR IEP DEVELOPMENT

In accordance with Public Law 94-142, the social worker has an assigned role in the IEP process after the appropriate assessments have been conducted. He or she serves as a liaison between the parent and the school system to ensure parental involvement in all facets of assessment and related service delivery. This function is critical, in that a major purpose of the IEP process is to serve as a vehicle for communication between the parents and the school about the child's education.

In addition, the social worker serves as a resource for the school's multidisciplinary team. Information is often needed by educators about the parents and the family dynamics (for example, specific information regarding the family composition and the child's relationship with parents and siblings). The social worker, who is trained in group dynamics, can function in this role of promoting effective communication while ensuring parent's rights.

ISSUES, CONCERNS, AND RECOMMENDATIONS

Numerous factors serve as barriers to the effective implementation of Public Law 94-142, particularly those related to social work services. Conceptually, these factors will be differentiated as those internal to the profession that the profession can somewhat readily affect, and those external to or outside the profession. Recommendations are offered that could promote the effective service delivery by social workers to handicapped children.

External Factors

Human service providers have traditionally cited inadequate funding as a critical impediment in the delivery of comprehensive services. Recent research findings related to school social work vis-à-vis Public Law 94-142 also document such a problem (Levine, 1984). It has been found that fiscal constraints limit the availability of program options and cause substantial staffing problems. Social workers in large school systems frequently report that their time is almost solely spent trying to respond to the substantial number of requests for psychosocial (social history) assessments as required by law. It was learned in a meeting with a senior staff associate of the National Association of Social Workers (NASW) that the problem of social workers serving largely as "sociometrists" is also indicative of what may be transpiring on a national level (Hare, 1985).

Internal Factors

Because school administrators (principals) basically determine the climate or set the tone of a given program, it is critical that social workers develop strategies for providing information regarding what they can offer, particularly on a policy or program development level (Tabb, 1984). A prevalent problem of social work has been and continues to be "the selling of the profession"; clarifying concisely what it is social workers do, separate from other human service professions, and communicating that information to persons who affect the utilization and deployment of social workers. In a sense, good public relations needs to be an inherent part of social work practice so that the specialized skills and knowledge of its practitioners can be optimally utilized.

Also related to fiscal staffing constraints is the need for the profession to commit itself to determining service delivery options by way of additional research, and to attempts at innovative and, when necessary, nontraditional strategies for assisting clients or client groups.

Much of the burden for preparing social workers to overcome those identified barriers to implementation rests within those institutions responsible for training them. Critical areas viewed as necessary in the preparation of school social workers include coursework and training in the area of effective performance within organizations. When one is not majoring in administration, which most practitioners do not, little required formal training is available in the areas of organizational analysis and development. As noted earlier, very often it is a system's structure and policies that may adversely affect a client or client group. In such cases, intervention may be most appropriate at the organizational level rather than at the traditional casework or clinical level.

Additionally, professional schools of social work should give practitioners a more thorough background in appropriate or relevant legislation. Social work students who have identified their interest area as working with children should have some preparatory knowledge of juvenile law and laws pertaining to child abuse and neglect. Practitioners interested in school social work should also have a working knowledge of relevant school laws such as compulsory school attendance. It is equally imperative that school social workers have a basic knowledge of Public Law 94-142 and related state bylaws, in order to develop services consistent with those mandated.

Schools of social work education have the important responsibility of providing practitioners with the necessary knowledge and skills in areas affecting children in schools, specifically special education. One of the school social worker's major responsibilities is the dissemination, interpretation, and, at times, implementation of such legal requirements in ways that effectively help both children and their parents.

REFERENCES

Anderson, R. J. (1977). Implication for the practice of social work and the Education For All Handicapped Children Act. In National Association of Social Workers (Ed.), *NASW—School social work and P.L. 94-142. The Education For All Handicapped Children Act* (pp. 91–98). Washington, D.C.: National Association of Social Workers, Inc.

Byrne, J. L., Hare, I., Hooper, S. N., Morse, B. J., & Sabatino, C. A. (1977). The role of a social history in special education evaluation. In National Association of Social Workers (Ed.), *NASW—School social work and P.L. 94-142. The Education For All Handicapped Children Act* (pp. 47–55). Washington, D.C.: National Association of Social Workers, Inc.

Education of the Handicapped Regulations. (1985). 34 Code of Federal Regulations Part 300, Supplement 138.

Gallant, C. B. (1982). *Mediation in special education disputes.* Maryland: The National Association of Social Workers, Inc.

Hare, I. (7 Oct. 1985). Interview. Silver Spring, MD: National Association of Social Workers.

Levine, R. S. (1984). Barriers to the implementation of P.L. 94-142. *Social Work in Education, 7*(1), 22–34.

National Association of Social Workers. (Ed.) (1977). *NASW—School Social Work and P.L. 94-142. The Education For All Handicapped Children Act.* Washington, D.C.: National Association of Social Workers, Inc.

Oppenheimer, J. J. (1925). *The visiting teacher movement, with special reference to administrative relationships* (2nd ed.). Rochester, NY: Joint Committee on Methods of Preventing Delinquency.

Tabb, S. M. (1984). *The organizational climate of public schools: A human services approach.* Unpublished doctoral dissertation, University of Maryland, College Park.

Virginia State Board of Education (1977). Superintendent's memo #6355, June 2, 1972. In National Association of Social Workers (Ed.). (1977). *NASW—School Social Work and P.L. 94-142. The Education For All Handicapped Children Act.* Washington, D.C.: National Association of Social Workers, Inc.

Wilkerson, W. W. (1977). Administrative requirements and guidelines for special education programs. In National Association of Social Workers (Ed.), *NASW— School social work and P.L. 94-142. The Education For All Handicapped Children Act* (pp. 47–48). Washington, D.C.: National Association of Social Workers, Inc.

Chapter **14**

Speech Pathology

Shiela Applestein

The role of the speech therapist has traditionally been to provide speech correction services to school-age children on an itinerant basis. With the passage of Public Law 94-142, the speech therapist's role was expanded to include speech and language services. Today, the American Speech-Language-Hearing Association recommends the use of the term speech-language pathologist.

DEFINITION OF SPEECH PATHOLOGY

Speech pathology services have been defined in the Public Law 94-142 Regulations as follows:

(i)   Identification of children with speech or language disorders;
(ii) Diagnosis and appraisal of specific speech or language disorders;
(iii) Referral for medical or other professional attention necessary for the habilitation of speech or language disorders;
(iv) Provisions of speech and language services for the habilitation or prevention of communicative disorders; and
(v)   Counseling and guidance of parents, children, and teachers regarding speech and language disorders. (Education of the Handicapped Regulations, 1985)

The classification "speech impaired," as used in Public Law 94-142 and changed to the classification "speech or language impaired" in Public Law 98-199 (Sec. 2(1)), comprises children with communication disorders, such as stuttering, impaired articulation, a language impairment, or a voice impairment, which adversely affect the children's educational performance (EHLR Special Report, 1984).

Formal definitions for communication disorders which include speech and language disorders have been adopted by the American Speech-Language-Hearing Association (1982).

Speech disorders are as follows:

Voice disorder—the absence or abnormal production of vocal quality, pitch, loudness, resonance, or duration.

Articulation disorder—the abnormal production of speech sounds.

Fluency disorder—the impairment of rate and rhythm of the flow of verbal expression, which may be accompanied by struggle behavior.

Language disorders involve the impairment or deviant development of comprehension or use of any of the following aspects of language:

Phonology—the sound system of a language and the linguistic rules that govern the sound combinations.

Morphology—the linguistic system that governs the structure of words and the construction of word forms from the basic elements of meaning.

Syntax—the linguistic rule governing the order and combination of words to form sentences, and the relationships among the elements within a sentence.

Semantics—the psycholinguistic system that patterns the content of an utterance, intent, and meanings of words and sentences.

Pragmatics—the sociolinguistic system that patterns the use of language in communication, which may be expressed motorically, vocally, or verbally.

A communicative difference that reflects regional, social, or cultural/ethnic factors should not be considered a disorder of speech or language. A communicative disorder may result in a primary handicapping condition or may be secondary to other documented handicapping conditions.

RELATIONSHIP TO SPECIAL EDUCATION

Speech pathology services may be classified as special education or as related services under federal law and regulations, as shown in Table 14–1. Although states have been given the option to define speech pathology services as a related service only, not one state has chosen to do so. The probable reason is that such a change might have an adverse impact on the

Table 14–1. Classification of Speech Pathology Services as Special Education or Related Services Under Federal Regulations

	Special Education	Related Services
Eligibility	Primary handicapping condition is speech or language impairment	Primary handicapping condition may be speech or language impairment. Communicative disorder may be secondary to another handicapping condition.
Services offered	Speech pathology services are the only instructional services offered to meet the needs of the handicapped child	Speech pathology services are supportive services offered to assist the handicapped child to benefit from special education services provided (i.e., a class for the language-impaired, hearing-impaired, or mentally retarded)

Public Law 94-142 funding that would be available for service delivery (Dublinske and Healey, 1978).

The provision of speech pathology services to children who do not have problems in academic performance has been an ongoing issue related to Public Law 94-142 regulations. A policy interpretation of the term "adversely affects academic performance" as it relates to speech- or language-impaired children was made by Edwin Martin, former Assistant Secretary in the Office of Special Education and Rehabilitative Services in the Department of Education, in a 1980 letter to Stanley Dublinske. This interpretation suggested that a child who is handicapped because of a speech or language impairment cannot be denied service because there are no concomitant academic problems. Martin stated, "The extent of a child's mastery of the basic skill of effective oral communication is clearly includable within the standard of 'educational performance' set by the regulations. Therefore, a speech/language impairment necessarily adversely affects educational performance when the communication disorder is judged sufficiently severe to require the provision of speech-pathology services to the child . . . [. T]he determination of the child's status as a 'handicapped child' cannot be conditioned on a requirement that there be a concurrent deficiency in academic performance."

This interpretation provides clarification of "educational performance" to include both academic performance and psychosocial competencies as they relate to effective oral communication. Therefore, children who have no apparent academic problems but who exhibit language, articulation, voice, or fluency disorders may be considered handicapped and eligible to receive services under Public Law 94-142.

ELIGIBILITY FOR RELATED SERVICE PROVISION

Speech-language pathologists are the qualified examiners for the handicapping condition speech- or language-impaired. They have the primary responsibility for the assessment of children who are suspected of having communicative disorders characterized by language deficits that may be the basis for academic difficulties, articulation disorders, chronic voice disorders, and fluency disorders. Speech and language disorders associated with other conditions, such as hearing impairment, cleft palate, cerebral palsy, intellectual limitation, and emotional disturbance, are also assessed.

The composition of the multidisciplinary team for the assessment of a handicapped child, as required by Public Law 94-142 regulations, must include at least one member with expertise in the area of the suspected disability. For children with a speech impairment, a team composed of the speech-language pathologist and the child's regular classroom teacher would meet the Public Law 94-142 requirements. Additional specialists, such as a psychologist or diagnostic teacher, may be included in the assessment team designated for children suspected of having language disorders (Dublinske and Healey, 1978).

A clinical evaluation is needed to establish diagnosis and extent of impairment, in order to confirm or rule out a communicative disorder as a handicapping condition (Turnbull, Strickland, and Brantley, 1978). This evaluation should utilize both formal and informal assessment procedures that are appropriate for the communicatively handicapped child as determined by the speech-language pathologist. Local school districts, in interpreting evaluation data and making placement decisions, are responsible for using information from a variety of sources, including aptitude and achievement tests, teacher recommendations, physical condition, social or cultural background, and adaptive behavior. A complete battery of assessments (psychological or achievement testing) is not required for children who have a speech or language impairment as their primary handicapping condition (Education of the Handicapped Regulations, 1985). The speech-language pathologist, however, may recommend referrals for additional assessments needed to make an appropriate diagnosis or placement decision. The multisource requirement is clarified in relation to speech or language impaired children in the comment following Federal Regulations 300.533. "While all the named sources would have to be used for a child whose suspected disability is mental retardation, they would not be necessary for certain other handicapped children, such as a child who has a severe articulation disorder as his or her primary handicap. For such a child, the speech-language pathologist, in complying with the multi-source requirement, might use (1) a standardized test of articulation and (2) observation of the child's articulation behavior in conversational speech" (Education of the Handicapped Regulations, 1985).

Reports based upon the evaluation have no required format but must address the child's strengths and weaknesses and include a statement of services shown to be needed by the assessment data. Although Federal regulations supply general criteria for the classification of speech or language impaired children, it is the responsibility of each state to determine the specific criteria by which eligibility for speech pathology services is determined (Turnbull et al., 1978). Several states and local education agencies have established criteria for such services designating levels of impairment from severe to mild. Some speech and language tests have a severity rating as part of the test scores.

For a child with a suspected speech or language impairment who is being considered for placement in special education, no specific person must represent the evaluation team at the placement meeting. However, the public agency must ensure that either a member of the evaluation team or a person knowledgeable about the evaluation procedures used and familiar with the results of the evaluation participate in the meeting. For a child whose primary handicap is a speech or language impairment, the speech-language pathologist would normally be the appropriate representative participating in the placement meeting (Education of the Handicapped Regulations, 1985). A state or local education agency may impose requirements that are less flexible or more stringent than those mandated by federal law in determining team composition.

OPTIONS IN SERVICE DELIVERY MODELS

Service delivery models in schools must provide a continuum of services appropriate to meet the needs of the communicatively handicapped child in the least restrictive environment. The American Speech-Language-Hearing Association (1984) recommends that an appropriate model of service delivery be determined through the evaluation process and the application of severity criteria. Although the severity of the disorder is a prime consideration in determining which services are needed to meet the goals and objectives of the IEP, other factors must be considered: (1) the impact of the communication disorder on the child's ability to function in an academic setting; (2) the relationship of the communication disorder(s) to other handicapping conditions; (3) the stage of development of the communication disorder; and (4) other factors related to the individual child's needs.

Four types of delivery models are recommended by the American Speech-Language-Hearing Association to be utilized as guidelines in developing a comprehensive service delivery model for communicatively handicapped children in the schools. The speech-language pathologist is the primary person responsible for the development, management, coordination, and evaluation of the programs described. Consideration is given to whether the service is provided directly by the speech-language pathologist, indirectly through the classroom teacher, parent(s), or supportive personnel, or with the assistance of modules or self-paced programs. Consideration is also given in the resource room and self-contained programs as to who is the primary provider of the child's academic instruction: the speech-language pathologist, the classroom teacher, or both. The service delivery models described are the consultation program, the itinerant program, the resource room program, and the self-contained program.

Successful programs will integrate these four models and, in some instances use a combination of models to best meet the individual needs of children. A speech-language pathologist may provide intensive therapy to a group of severe-profound children using the resource room model and work with the remainder of his or her caseload using the itinerant model. By developing delivery models based upon these guidelines, options will be available to ensure that communicatively impaired children are educated in the least restrictive environment.

Consultation Program (Indirect Service)

This program is suitable for all disorders and ranges of severity. The speech-language pathologist develops a clinical management program for the child and is responsible for training and instructing others to carry it out. The speech-language pathologist does not work directly with the child (other than for assessment and demonstration). Teachers, parents, and supportive personnel are trained in methods of intervention and provide the direct service to the child. This model gives the speech-language pathologist an opportunity to fill a new and emerging role as consultant in the schools. The consultation model may be used in a variety of ways:

To review a child's progress after dismissal from direct service
To provide intensive language stimulation in the natural environment for children who are severely/profoundly mentally handicapped or multiply-handicapped
To provide consultation services to children who have mild communicative disorders
To assist parents and staff members in understanding a child's communication difficulties

Children seen on a consultative basis may be included in the annual child count.

Itinerant Program (Intermittent Direct Service)

This program is the traditional model historically used by speech-language pathologists. Children identified as mildly to severely impaired are placed in regular or special classrooms and are seen for speech-pathology services in addition to their academic program. Children may leave their classrooms, or the speech-language pathologist may provide service to the children within their classrooms. The teacher has the primary responsibility for the child's academic program; however, the speech-language pathologist attempts to incorporate academic content into the service program. Goals and objectives are more likely to be attained when educators are involved in reinforcement of the intervention plan within the educational setting. Children in the itinerant program are given direct service either individually or in small groups for the habilitation of speech and language disorders.

Resource Room Program (Intensive Direct Service)

This program is designed to serve children with severe communication disorders. It is typically used for articulation and language disorders but is suited for all classifications of disorders. In addition to receiving direct service from the speech-language pathologist individually or in a small group, the child may be involved with self-paced instruction selected and prepared by the speech-language pathologist that addresses specific deficit areas. The speech-language pathologist also cooperates with the regular or special education teacher by incorporating communication skill–building activities into the child's total curriculum. The classroom teacher has primary responsibility for academic instruction, and the speech-language pathologist incorporates academic curriculum into the resource room program.

Self-Contained Program (Academically Integrated Direct Service)

This program is a self-contained program for children who have severe or multiple communicative disorders and whose needs will be ideally met by a speech-language pathologist. Children placed in this type of setting have primary educational/social needs in the area of communication, regardless of etiology. Academic instruction is provided by the speech-language pathologist. State education agencies may require that a speech-language pathologist be certified in another area of education, or the speech-language pathologist may team with a certified classroom teacher in order to implement this model within state guidelines.

IMPLICATIONS FOR IEP DEVELOPMENT

The IEP developed for a child identified as speech- or language-impaired must include all of the components as required by Public Law 94-142 regulations related to developing an individualized education program. If a child is receiving speech pathology services, the federal regulations indicate that the child's teacher could be the speech-language pathologist for the purpose of the IEP meeting. Another speech-language pathologist, a special education teacher, or a supervisor could serve as the representative of the public agency (Education of the Handicapped Regulations, 1985).

If a child has an identified need for speech pathology services as a related service, the speech-language pathologist could either attend the meeting or otherwise be involved in developing the IEP. A written recommendation concerning the nature, frequency, and amount of service recommended should be provided if the related services personnel are not represented at the meeting. If a child is receiving other special education services because of a primary handicapping condition, the special education teacher would attend the meeting as the child's teacher.

The IEP for the speech- or language-impaired child should focus on improving the child's communication skills by either correcting the impairment or minimizing its effect on the child's ability to communicate. It must include a statement indicating the frequency of sessions per week and the approximate duration of each session. All services the child needs as determined by the current evaluation, regardless of availability to the public agency, must be included in the IEP (Rules and Regulations, 1981). If it is agreed at the IEP development meeting that special materials, equipment, or aids are needed for a communicatively handicapped child, these should be listed on the IEP.

The IEP for the child receiving speech pathology services is reviewed at least annually, as is required by Public Law 94-142 regulations for all handicapped children. By writing instructional objectives in such a manner as to include "when" the objective is to be accomplished and the "criterion" level, the speech-language pathologist can initiate the review using the method cited in the objective. The evaluation will determine whether the child has met the criterion level and accomplished the "what" indicated in the objective (Dublinske, 1978).

ISSUES, CONCERNS, AND RECOMMENDATIONS

Federal and state legislation and local education agency interpretations of the legislation have had a significant impact on the functional role of the speech-language pathologist in the schools. Modification and expansion of the speech-language pathologist's role as a part of the total service delivery process have raised many issues related to the delivery of appropriate speech pathology services in schools (Blanchard and Nober, 1978).

Some states have equated the terms "educational performance" and "academic achievement," an interpretation that may lead to denial of services to children otherwise eligible to receive them. Increased paperwork, available service delivery models, entry and exit criteria, severity indices, minimum and maximum caseloads, and staff development need to be addressed at state and local levels to ensure that appropriate speech pathology services can continue to be provided to identified speech- or language-impaired children.

A serious problem facing many school districts is the insufficient number of speech-language pathologists employed to meet the needs of speech-impaired children. Because of this staffing shortage, school districts will have to develop a variety of innovative service delivery models for children in elementary, middle, junior high, and senior high schools. They will also need to consider the age of onset of the child's speech or language problem as well as other concomitant handicapping conditions.

Dublinske (1978) notes that speech-language pathologists have traditionally developed individualized programs for children with speech or language disorders. The Public Law 94-142 regulations require that these activities be completed within specified times, documented in written form, and subjected to uniform procedures. If the IEP is properly designed and used as it was intended, with measurable objectives and good evaluation criteria, speech-language pathologists are in a better position to evaluate and restructure services when necessary, thereby having the opportunity to improve the quality and quantity of services to communicatively handicapped children.

REFERENCES

American Speech-Language-Hearing Association. Committee on language, speech and hearing services in the schools. (1982). Definition: Communicative disorders and variations. *ASHA, 24*(11), 949–950.

American Speech-Language-Hearing Association. Committee on language, speech and hearing services in the schools. (1984). Guidelines for caseload size for speech-language services in the schools. *ASHA, 26*(4), 53-58.

Blanchard, M. M. & Nober, E. H. (1978). The impact of state and federal legislation on public school speech, language and hearing clinicians. *Language, Speech and Hearing Services in Schools, 9*(2), 77–84.

Dublinske, S. (1978). Public Law 94-142: Developing the individualized education program (IEP). *ASHA, 20*(5), 380–397.

Dublinske, S., & Healey, W. C. (1978). Public Law 94-142: Questions and answers for the speech-language pathologist and audiologist. *ASHA, 20*(3), 188–205.

Education of the Handicapped Regulations. (1985). 34 Code of Federal Regulations Part 300, Supplement 138.

EHLR Special Report: Amendments of EHA by Public Law 98-199, Supplement 112 (1984).

Rules and Regulations for Public Law 94-142. (1981, January 19). *Federal Register, 46.*

Turnbull, A. P., Strickland, B., & Brantley, J. C. (1978). *Developing and implementing individualized education programs.* Columbus, OH: Charles E. Merrill.

Chapter 15

Transportation

Linda F. Bluth

In accordance with Public Law 94-142, transportation is required to be provided as a related service if a child has been identified as handicapped, and the handicapping condition requires placement in a school to which the child needs transportation in order to receive special education services.

DEFINITION OF TRANSPORTATION

Transportation, as defined in Public Law 94-142, consists of

(i)   Travel to and from school and between schools;
(ii) Travel in and around school buildings; and
(iii) Specialized equipment (such as special or adapted buses, lifts and ramps), if required to provide special transportation for a handicapped child.
(Education of the Handicapped Regulations, 1985)

Transportation of handicapped children is an important consideration in relationship to special education accessibility. Many handicapped children with a variety of handicapping conditions are capable of using the same transportation services as non-handicapped children; however, other, more severely handicapped children require specialized transportation services, such as lift buses that can accommodate wheelchairs. Appropriate decision-making regarding transportation is therefore essential to providing special education to handicapped children (Bluth, 1985a).

Because special transportation service is the most visible of all related services, it receives attention from school board members, community leaders, administrators, and parents. Therefore, each local educational district must have adequate written transportation policies and procedures that are in compliance with federal and individual state mandates. Careful analyses of a district's unique situations are essential in order to establish sound practices in delivery of service.

In addition to Public Law 94-142, Section 504 of Public Law 93-112, passed by Congress as part of the Rehabilitation Act of 1973, requires that "No otherwise qualified handicapped individual in the United States . . . shall solely by reason of his handicap be excluded from participation in, be denied the benefits of, or be subjected to discrimination under any program or activity receiving Federal financial assistance" (Vocational Rehabilitation Act of 1973).

Section 504 of Public Law 93-112 defines free education as the provision of educational and related services without cost to handicapped persons or to their parents or guardians, except for those fees that are imposed on non-handicapped persons or their parents or guardians. Part of the Transportation portion reads as follows:

> If a recipient places a handicapped person in or refers such person to a program not operated by the recipient as its means of carrying out the requirements of this subpart, the recipient shall ensure that adequate transportation to and from the program is provided at no greater cost than would be incurred by the person or his or her parents or guardian if the person were placed in the program operated by the recipient. (Public Law 93-112)

For example, if a child is identified as seriously emotionally disturbed and requires the related service transportation for access to his or her assigned public school program, and the local school district and parent are in agreement to a change of placement in a school out of the district, the parent cannot be required to pay for transportation costs.

RELATIONSHIP TO SPECIAL EDUCATION

The interpretation of the meaning of transportation as a related service under Public Law 94-142 varies. Bluth (1985b) has recommended the following guidelines:

1. If a child has not been designated eligible for special education, there can be no related service determination. Student transportation provisions are therefore not covered for these children under Public Law 94-142 or Public Law 93-112.
2. If a child is identified as needing special education and the related service transportation, this service must be provided without cost to the parent, guardian, or child.
3. The need for special education does not automatically authorize the provision of the related service transportation. Authorization is an IEP committee's decision.

4. Each transportation service need is required to be examined independently by an IEP committee. Individual school district policies must be developed in conformance with federal and state mandates. Policies and procedures should be in writing and provided to all required parties, to ensure compliance with standards for implementation of transportation services.

Because the transportation needs of handicapped children vary from child to child, local education agencies have had to develop written guidelines for the provision of this related service. The following typical situations described by Bluth (1985b) are suggested for inclusion in a district's written guidelines pertaining to the transportation of handicapped children:

If an orthopedically impaired child lives within the prescribed walking distance to a school, but because of the specific nature of the handicapping condition, the child cannot safely reach the school, then the child requires the related service transportation.

If a seriously emotionally disturbed child has been suspended from a school to which he or she previously walked and is now being sent to a school beyond the prescribed walking distance, the child now needs transportation as a related service, and the IEP committee must be convened in order to include this service in the IEP.

If a child is determined no longer to require school bus transportation, the IEP committee must meet to remove this related service from the IEP.

ELIGIBILITY FOR RELATED SERVICE PROVISION

Because of the many different considerations (for example, child's independent functioning level, severity of the handicapped condition, location of school), it is essential that state and local education agencies provide written guidelines for IEP committee members to ensure consistent decision-making about transportation issues. In addition, each local education agency should identify the representative of the public agency who is qualified to make recommendations to the IEP committee regarding the related service transportation and can address this area in the IEP meeting. It is essential to delegate to this individual the authority to make individual case determinations in accordance with Public Laws 94-142 and 93-112.

The determination that a child who is handicapped needs transportation as a related service must be made by someone qualified to make the decision. Such a person might be a special educator, a physical therapist, or a psychologist. The input of transportation personnel is also essential in order to facilitate the safest and most efficient method of service delivery.

OPTIONS IN SERVICE DELIVERY MODELS

The service model options for each of the handicapping conditions must be carefully considered. Some children may require very specialized services, while others may not require the related service. The majority of handicapped children, however, require special related service transportation because of school placement site, child's age, or special needs (Bluth, 1985b).

Deaf.   Deaf children most often require special transportation services because of the distant location of their school placement. It is essential that transporters of this population be familiar with these children's mode of communication. If the primary mode of communication is sign language, it should be identified as such in the IEP. Transporters of this population may require training in special communication techniques in order to facilitate rapport and safety.

Deaf-Blind.   Children with concomitant hearing and visual impairments require special transportation considerations to ensure safety, to maximize mobility considerations, and to accommodate special communication needs. The transporters need very specialized training in working with these children.

Hard of Hearing.   The transportation service needs of a hard-of-hearing child are often determined by the school placement location. The transporters should receive in-service training in sign language and other communication techniques to enhance the children's safety and rapport.

Mentally Retarded.   Because mentally retarded children range in ability and functioning level, some (mildly and moderately retarded) do not require special transportation services because of their independent functioning level and appropriate adaptive skills. Severely and profoundly mentally retarded children often require special transportation services because of their needs and dependent functioning level. The determination of the need for this special service is often based upon independent functioning level, child safety factors, and school location.

Multihandicapped.   Children with multiple handicaps often require carefully planned transportation services because of the seriousness of their handicapping condition. The combination of handicaps requires specialized group decision-making by all relevant persons (special educators, related services providers, agencies, and parents).

Orthopedically Impaired.   Orthopedically impaired children also require individually planned transportation services. Some children can use regular transportation vehicles, but other children require lift buses and very specially developed adapted equipment. The transporters of this population need specialized training in appropriate adaptive equipment management as well as in special handling of school bus equipment.

Other Health-Impaired.   This very broad category includes children with limited strength, vitality, or alertness due to chronic or acute health problems. They may utilize the regular school bus or may require special transportation. The driver of this population should be adequately informed about the specific health impairments and the special transportation considerations required.

Seriously Emotionally Disturbed.   Seriously emotionally disturbed children may or may not require special transportation, depending upon school location and transportation behavior. In extreme cases, a special bus aide is essential to manage children's behavior and ensure their safety. These children's transportation needs should be carefully addressed in each IEP. The transporters of this population are in need of extensive behavior management training.

Specific Learning Disabled.   Children with specific learning disabilities rarely require special school bus transportation unless they are attending a special school.

Speech-Impaired.   Speech-impaired children usually do not require special school transportation.

Visually Impaired.   Children with visual impairments may or may not require special transportation, depending on level of independent functioning and location of school. Some children may require assistance when moving about the school bus, and some may need a special seat assignment in order to maximize safety.

IMPLICATIONS FOR IEP DEVELOPMENT

After the IEP committee has determined that a child is eligible for transportation as a related service, the individualized education program (IEP) is the instrument for recording the child's transportation services. This document is where all the child's services are recorded. It provides for both accountability and control of delivery of service agreement.

Transportation should be defined in the IEP to the extent that this service is provided in a manner that is unique and exceeds transportation requirements for nonhandicapped children. This need can be recorded under "annual goals," including short-term objectives. The frequency of this service, and all special delivery of service modifications (lift bus, assistive harness device, special helmet) should be specified in writing. All information about a given child should be recorded in the IEP and approved prior to actual implementation. The IEP must be signed by the IEP committee of which the parent or guardian is a member. If there is a dispute or a parent or guardian is dissatisfied with the determination of the type of transportation services recommended by the IEP committee, the parent has the right to request an impartial due process hearing in accordance with federal and state provisions.

The IEP committee should always recommend transportation services most appropriate to the individual child's need. A child in a wheelchair who is in need of a lift bus cannot be excluded from school because the school district does not have this equipment available. Written guidelines in compliance with federal and state mandates should be disseminated by special education and transportation departments as a joint effort to facilitate decision-making for the IEP committee. If the committee approves recreation after school hours as a related service, then transportation must be provided to facilitate this service. When an extended school year is approved as part of the IEP, such approval is a condition of the IEP, and transportation must be free and in accordance with the regular school year practices.

One of the most questioned areas has been a district's responsibility for transportation when the district has chosen a residential facility for the child. School districts are responsible for travel to and from the residential placement. The number of round trips should be determined by the IEP committee. Some states provide between three and four round trips annually. If a residential facility requires home visits on a more frequent basis, this consideration should be specified in the IEP prior to placement.

Each school district must determine at what age it is safe to initiate transportation services for handicapped children to receive special education services. This is a very important consideration for states mandating services beginning at birth. Vehicle selection and adequate supervision are important IEP considerations in developing special education service recommendations.

Transportation planning and services require coordination between special education and transportation departments. Each of these departments must clearly define its respective responsibilities to provide the related service of transportation. Written guidelines, policies, and procedures, as well as required forms, must meet the needs of both departments. An IEP meeting must be conducted at least annually for the purpose of reviewing and, if appropriate, revising recommended services. Under federal regulations, there can be no undue delay in providing related services to children in special education.

The method of transportation service delivery is not specified in Public Law 94-142. Each state has individual guidelines for this area. Specific state guidelines may determine how a local education agency can accommodate handicapped children's transportation needs. Some options are (1) owning the transportation vehicles, (2) contracting transportation services, (3) renting transportation vehicles, (4) sharing ownership of vehicles, and (5) reimbursing a private carrier or parent/guardian for transportation costs.

Vehicle choice is not specified in Public Law 94-142 or Public Law 93-112. This determination is made by each local education agency. According to Public Law 94-142, "specialized equipment (such as special or adapted buses, lift and ramps), if required to provide special transportation for a handicapped child," should be provided to assure appropriate transportation. Handicapped students can be transported on any of a variety of vehicles that comply with individual state laws and the local school district's policies. A standard school bus, a school bus with adapted equipment, mass transit system services (bus or subway), minibus, van unit, taxi cab, or private vehicle may be used.

It is appropriate for the choice of vehicle to be recommended by the IEP committee and recorded in the IEP. Matters of liability regarding vehicle choice should be defined by the individual school district and presented to all concerned parties in writing (Bluth, 1985a).

ISSUES, CONCERNS, AND RECOMMENDATIONS

The following transportation issues have received attention as a result of the passage of Public Law 94-142.

Transportation Costs

Transportation is to be provided at no charge to a handicapped child if this related service is required for the child to benefit from special education. Insufficient transportation funds is never an acceptable reason for not providing a handicapped child with transportation services.

If a local school system approves the placement of a handicapped child in a program it does not operate, it must ensure that transportation is provided at no cost to the parent. When the school system and parent agree that the parent will transport the child to a public or nonpublic school, that agreement must provide for reimbursement of the parent. Public Laws 94-142 and 93-112 do not set a reimbursement schedule. Most state and local education agencies use travel reimbursement schedules to determine the amount of the payment. General cost issues should be worked out prior to initiating service delivery. If the parent and the school system do not agree on the adequacy of the reimbursement allowance, the dispute could be resolved by a due process hearing.

No parent or guardian is required to provide the related service of transportation. It is the obligation of an educational agency to provide transportation for a handicapped child regardless of a parent or guardian's inability or unwillingness to furnish transportation. The school system should have procedures to assure that parents providing transportation services have a valid license and meet individual state insurance provisions.

For a handicapped child placed in a distant residential facility for educational purposes, Public Law 94-142 does not set a standard for the number of allowed trips home. At minimum, most school systems provide transportation at the beginning and end of the school term and for scheduled school holidays or recesses. It is the responsibility of individual state or local education agencies to have written procedures or policies applying to this area. The number of trips home should be stated in the child's IEP.

Length of the Ride

Neither Public Law 94-142 nor Public Law 93-112 discusses a maximum travel time to transport handicapped children in order to obtain special education services. This matter should be addressed by state and local education agencies. The length of the ride should be determined on an individual basis and reviewed by the IEP committee.

As a general rule, transportation routing for a child should be limited to one hour each way whenever feasible. However, with parental knowledge and IEP committee approval, transportation travel may exceed this recommended time period if required by (1) distance of the home from the assigned school, (2) severity of the handicapping condition (possibly necessitating a distant school placement), (3) rush hour traffic in urban areas, (4) type of handicapping condition or (5) other unique situations requiring special arrangements. It is in the best interest of handicapped children that flexibility be provided for in determining length of the ride.

Location of Pickup and Drop-Off Points

Public Laws 94-142 and 93-112 do not establish requirements regarding pickup and drop-off locations. Local education agencies are responsible for picking up handicapped children at the residence of their parents or guardian unless prior alternative arrangements are mutually agreed upon. In addition, parents or guardians are responsible for bringing the handicapped child to the drive or curbside for pickup and for meeting the vehicle at the end of the school day at the drop-off point. Deviations due to individual circumstances must be agreed upon on an individual basis and noted in the IEP.

Each school district must have a written policy relating to pickup and drop-off practices, including how to respond to a situation when no authorized person is available to receive a child.

Location of loading and unloading sites for children with handicapping conditions may require alterations from standard operating procedures. These alterations should be noted in the IEP.

Disputes

Disputes regarding transportation cost, length of the ride, and location of pickup and drop-off points can be resolved through a due process hearing if agreement cannot be reached by a parent and school district.

Transportation Disciplinary and Suspension Procedures for Handicapped Students

Handicapped children, like nonhandicapped children, are subject to disciplinary action(s) pursuant to the written rules of state and local education agencies. The issue of school bus disciplinary or suspension action requires an IEP committee review, because transportation is provided as a related service. In accordance with Public Law 93-112, no handicapped child may be subjected to punitive action solely on the basis of the handicap. The problem that arises is the relationship between the proposed disciplinary action and the handicapping condition. When it appears that the behavior for which the child is to be removed from transportation service is the result of the child's handicapping condition, the child cannot be deprived of access to special education services. This is not to say that if the behavior is of danger to the driver and other children, transportation of the child may not be interrupted.

An interruption of transportation necessitates an emergency IEP meeting. It is recommended that when an interruption of this kind exceeds five school days, or a total of ten school days in a given school year, an IEP meeting be held. It is clear that a child cannot be suspended permanently from transportation services if this suspension prevents access to special education services. Such action is considered discriminatory and would violate Public Law 93-112. Specifically, for a suspension of transportation services in excess of five school days, the child and parents should be given procedural safeguards. If at an IEP meeting it is determined that the child's handicap was a significant cause of the behavior that prompted the disciplinary action, then the suspension should be rescinded.

In some extreme cases a change in educational placement to a more restrictive environment is required because of the severity of transportation problems. In most instances, however, additional supervisory staff or management strategies are successful in modifying the situation. Although Public Laws 94-142 and 93-112 do not directly address the question of suspension, school systems have begun to recognize the need to develop written procedures based upon court decisions, in order to address suspension issues equitably. Disputes about suspension of transportation services are subject to due process review under Public Law 94-142.

Emergencies

School bus drivers and aides should be familiar with the handicapped children they transport and the characteristics of their handicapping conditions. Knowledge about individual handicapped children prevents "over-identification" of what is or is not an emergency situation. Each school district must make provisions for emergency cards containing child's name, handicapping condition, and special transportation needs, to be carried on the school bus. It is recommended that parents complete an emergency card annually and give approval for the use of this information. All information should be handled as confidential data under the Family Educational Rights and Privacy Act of 1974, also known as the Buckley Amendment. This act covers all records, files, documents, and other materials that contain information directly relating to a child. Both the maintenance and use of emergency information should be in accord with federal, state, and local policies.

Evacuation Drills

It is essential to have a written plan for special emergency evacuations, with specific provisions for those children who use assistive devices and wheelchairs. Evacuation procedures should be well-known and rehearsed by drivers and aides to assure competent handling of both ambulatory and nonambulatory children in an emergency situation.

Handicapped children with physical, emotional, and mental limitations should be familiarized with evacuation procedures to their maximum capacity in a safe and organized manner. Whether handicapped children ride regular buses or specially adapted buses, they should be instructed to function within their individual capabilities. There should be a written plan to be followed and practiced with periodic drills. A written plan should include emergency stop locations, phone locations if there is no two-way radio system, and charted (shortest) routes to the hospital(s).

It is suggested that a seating chart with children's photographs be available for nonverbal children. Photographs should also be attached to emergency cards. These provisions should be made in addition to the IEP services identified.

Further Recommendations

Beyond the requirements set forth in Public Law 94-142, additional special practices can facilitate efficiency in transporting handicapped children.

In addition to a school system's transportation manual, specific written guidelines should be provided to the drivers and aides to increase their understanding of handicapped children. These guidelines should contain information about Public Law 94-142 requirements; Public Law 93-112 (Section 504) requirements; characteristics of the handicapping conditions; IEP development, content approval, implementation; and due process.

Annual in-service training is recommended for drivers and aides, with instruction provided in IEP implementation, disciplinary procedures, communication skills, behavior management, seating management, schedule management, assistive devices management, emergency procedures, special evacuation procedures, and loading and unloading procedures.

All transportation personnel need to be knowledgeable about handicapping conditions and the special needs of the children they are required to serve. Examples of special skills to be developed are:

Establishing a daily routine
Functioning as a cooperative team
Being consistent and fair with rules
Minimizing the number of bus rules as far as safety permits
Making sure individual children have the capacity to understand rules
Managing time in an efficient and realistic manner
Communicating at the functioning level of the individual child
Showing interest and approval of appropriate behavior
Rewarding appropriate behavior with attention and praise
Handling problems consistent with the school behavior management program

Adherence to these practices will result in a minimum of transportation problems.

In extreme instances where problems persist, the IEP committee will need to meet to review problems that directly affect safety. The IEP committee may recommend some special arrangements, such as: late pickup and early drop-off on the route, special seating arrangements, special aide arrangements, and individual student contact. These modifications must be a part of the IEP document.

CONCLUSION

Given the importance of recognizing special transportation needs of handicapped children, it is the responsibility of all those involved in providing services to these children to fulfill their assigned roles in an effective and efficient manner. A successful transportation program is contingent upon the cooperative involvement of children, parents, transportation specialists, special education personnel, and the community.

REFERENCES

Bluth, L. (1985a). Transportation of handicapped students. *National School Bus Report, 18*(3), 26–27.

Bluth, L. (1985b). *Transporting handicapped students: A resource manual and recommended guidelines for school transportation and special education personnel.* Washington, D.C.: National Association of State Directors of Special Education.

Education of the Handicapped Regulations. (1985). 34 Code of Federal Regulations Part 300, Supplement 138.

PART III
RESOURCES

Suggested Readings

AIDS and herpes carry weighty policy implications for your Board. (1985, October). *American School Board Journal.*

American Speech-Language-Hearing Association. (1983). Audiology services in the schools—position statement. *ASHA, 25,* 53–60.

American Speech-Language-Hearing Association. Committee on language, speech and hearing services in the schools. (1983). Recommended service delivery models and caseload sizes for speech-language pathologists in the schools (draft). *ASHA, 25*(2), 65–70.

Beers, C. S., & Beers, J. W. (1980). Early identification of learning disabilities: Facts and fallacies. *Elementary School Journal, 81*(2), 67–76.

Bennett, C. W., & Runyan, C. M. (1982). Educators' perceptions of the effects of communication disorders upon educational performance. *Language, Speech and Hearing Services in Schools, 13,* 260–263.

Connolly, B., & Anderson, R. M. (1978). Severely handicapped children in the public schools: A new frontier for the physical therapist. *Physical Therapy, 58*(4), 433–438.

Education Law Reporter. (1985). St. Paul, MN: West Publishing Co., *21,* 447–453.

Fairchild, T. (1982). The school psychologist's role as an assessment consultant. *Psychology in the Schools, 19*(2), 200–208.

Fettner, A. G., & Cheek, W. A. (1985). *The truth about AIDS: Evolution of an epidemic.* NY: Holt, Rinehart and Winston.

Frasco, L. J. (1980). Health science for handicapped children in public schools: What does the law say? *Education Unlimited, 2*(3), 38–39.

Frassinelli, L., Superior, K., & Meyers, J. (1983). A consultation model for speech and language intervention. *ASHA, 25*(11), 25–30.

Gilfoyle, E., & Hays, C. (1979). Occupational therapy roles and functions in the education of the school-based handicapped student. *American Journal of Occupational Therapy, 33*(9), 565–576.

Jenkins, R. L. (1983, Winter). Mainstreaming, malpractice, and new roles for the school nurse. *Education, 104*(2), 206–212.

Krajewski, J. (1985, December). AIDS and the schools. *Counterpoint, 5*(1), 16.

Lichenstein, R. (1982). New instrument: Old problem for early identification. *Exceptional Children, 49*(1), 70–72.

Litigation and special education (special issue). (1986). *Exceptional Children, 52*(4).

Mawdsley, R. D. (1984). *Legal aspects of pupil transportation.* Topeka, KS: National Association on Legal Problems of Education.

Mitchell, M. M. & Lindsey, D. (1979). A model for establishing occupational therapy and physical therapy services in the public schools. *American Journal of Occupational Therapy, 33*(6), 361–364.

National Association of Social Workers. (1978). *Federal legislation and the school social worker.* (J. Evertts, Ed.). Washington, D.C.: National Association of Social Workers, Inc.

National Association of State School Nurse Consultants. (1982). PL 94-142— Education For All Handicapped Children Act of 1975. *Journal of School Health, 5*(8), 475–478.

Nicholson, C., & Alcorn, C. (1980). Educational applications of the WISC-R: A handbook of interpretive strategies and remedial recommendations. Los Angeles: Western Psychological Services.

Nutter, R. E. (1985). Counseling intervention used with exceptional students: A statewide assessment. *School Counselor, 32*(3), 224–230.

Regan, N. N. (1982). The implementation of occupational therapy services in rural school systems. *American Journal of Occupational Therapy, 36*(2), 85–89.

Schleifer, M. J., & Klein, S.D. (Eds.). (1981). Recreation and leisure. *Exceptional Parent, 11*(2), 21–29.

Sherman, S., & Robinson, N. (1982). *Ability testing of handicapped people: Dilemma for government, science, and the public.* Washington: National Academy Press.

U.S. Department of Education. Office of Special Education Services. (1984). Sixth Annual Report to Congress on the Implementation of Public Law 94-142: The Education of All Handicapped Children Act. Washington, D.C.: U.S. Government Printing office.

Sproles, H. H., Panther, E. E., & Lanier, J. E. (1978). PL 94–142 and its impact on the counselor's role. *Personnel and Guidance Journal, 57*(4), 210–212.

Steiner, L. (1983). Career counseling with the handicapped: The final stage: Some unique approaches. *Journal of Employment Counseling 20*(2), 73–80.

Wehman, P. (1980). Age appropriate recreation programs for the severely handicapped youth and adults. *Journal of the Association for the Severely Handicapped, 5*(4), 395–407.

Glossary

abnormal postures Neonatal reflexes persisting significantly beyond appropriate age level and interfering with the achievement of normal developmental milestones.

ambient noise Background noise present in any listening environment. Background noise is a product of a variety of sound sources, including equipment, climate control systems, and activities of other individuals in the vicinity of the environment.

amplification monitoring The process of providing daily listening checks and visual inspections of hearing aids and other amplification devices to ensure that they are in satisfactory working order.

anatomical correlates The parallel structure of the connections of the nerve cells.

attention deficit disorder (ADD) A term used by the American Psychiatric Association in 1980 to describe the behavioral characteristics of "hyperactivity" in children that were formerly called minimal brain dysfunction.

audiologist A nonmedical specialist who measures hearing levels and evaluates hearing defects.

audiometer An instrument used to measure hearing acuity. The measurement is usually recorded in decibels.

auditory training A method of teaching a hearing-impaired child to make full use of his or her hearing ability.

autism A severe disorder of communication and behavior.

behavioral model A model of intervention focusing on the observable behavior of a child and not on the cause of the behavior.

case management The management of a child's program by the disciplines responsible for special education and related services.

case manager The individual responsible for coordinating a child's program of special education and related services.

CAT scan An x-ray procedure that examines "slices" of the brain and produces exact pictures of the electrical output of the brain.

catheterization The insertion of a narrow rubber, plastic, metal, or glass tube into the body to empty the bladder or the kidneys.

central nervous system The integrating center for all bodily functions and behavior; it is composed of the brain and the spinal cord.

colostomy A surgical opening in the abdomen used for the elimination of solid waste matter from the body.

communicative difference/dialect A variation of a symbol system used by a group of individuals that reflects regional, social, or cultural factors. Variations or alterations in the use of a symbol system may be indicative of primary language interference and should not be considered a disorder of speech or language.

communication disorder A language or speech handicap.

due process hearing A hearing presided over by an impartial hearing officer to resolve an impasse between a school district and a parent so as to ensure that the constitutional rights of neither party are violated.

dycem A sheet of material placed on a table or other surface to increase friction and prevent sliding.

EEG Electroencephalogram; a method of measuring electrical activity in the brain.

EHA Education of all Handicapped Children Act of 1975, known as Public Law (PL) 94–142.

etiology The study of causes, reasons, or origins of disorders or diseases.

Federal Regulation 300 A definition and clarification of Public Law 94–142, the Education for All Handicapped Children Act of 1975.

fine motor activity An activity in which groups of small muscles are involved, such as writing or manipulating objects.

frequency chart A recording of the number of incidents of a specific behavior over a specified period.

gross motor activity An activity in which groups of large muscles are involved, such as running or jumping.

handling Using one's hands or other body parts to aid in directing and increasing a child's muscle tone while promoting the child's use of the most normal pattern possible.

holistic Emphasizing the wholeness of something.

impartial hearing officer (IHO) An individual appointed by a state department of education to preside over hearings at the local or state level.

individualized education program (IEP) A written plan of instruction for a handicapped child receiving special education and related services.

itinerant services Special education or related services provided to a child by a professional who travels to more than one school.

itinerant teacher A teacher or resource consultant who travels between schools or homes to teach or provide instructional materials to handicapped children.

least restrictive placement The concept of serving handicapped children in the most appropriate educational environment and to the maximum extent possible with nonhandicapped children.

lesion An abnormal change in the structure of an organ or tissue caused by disease or injury.

local education agency (LEA) A school district responsible for providing public school education through the twelfth grade.

low-incidence disabilities Handicapping conditions that are fewer or lower in number in comparison with other handicapping conditions (e.g., a combination of visual handicap and hearing impairment).

mainstreaming The concept of serving handicapped children in regular school programs with additional support personnel and supplemental services.

medical model A model of intervention focusing on the etiology or cause of a child's behavior or problem.

neurodevelopmental treatment (NDT) A form of physical therapeutic intervention used with neurologically impaired children that emphasizes inhibition of abnormal reflexes and facilitation of age appropriate reflexes and balance; also referred to as Bobath method.

neurological impairment A condition resulting from brain injury or malfunctioning of the central nervous system.

neurological substrate The underlying physical composition of the nervous system.

neurologist A medical doctor specializing in the diagnosis and treatment of the nervous system.

palpation An examiner's use of his or her fingers to determine the subjective quantity and quality of muscle tone, muscle bulk, and anatomical structure.

plateau A term used in special education to refer to a level of growth in learning at which a child no longer shows improvement.

positioning Using equipment and other devices to support a child's optimal body alignment, enabling the child to participate normally in functional activities; also used to help prevent or correct deformities.

posterior temporal area Left, rear part of the brain, which affects language development.

pre-motor area The front part of the brain, which controls motor functioning in the body.

projective test A personality test in which a child responds to unstructured materials such as pictures, ink blots, and incomplete sentences.

psychologist An individual qualified to evaluate and provide treatment in areas of mental functioning.

psychometrist An individual qualified to measure or evaluate psychological functioning through the use of intelligence tests.

psychotherapist An individual who treats mental disorders using psychological methods.

Public Law 94-142 The Education for all Handicapped Children Act of 1975, referred to also as EHA.

Public Law 98-199 The Education of the Handicapped Act Amendments of 1983.

range of motion (ROM) The maximum amount of motion, measured in degrees, that a joint allows a limb to move in a given direction.

reciprocal gait pattern The normal human bipedal pattern of walking.

residential facility A private or state-supported institution that provides a 24-hour educational, treatment, and care program.

residual hearing The "remaining" hearing that a hearing-impaired child may utilize.

Section 504 The last paragraph of Public Law 93-112, the Rehabilitation Act of 1973, which prohibits discrimination on the basis of handicap in all federally funded programs.

segregated special education day school A separate school only for handicapped children.

self-contained class A class taught for an entire school day by the same teacher; also called structured learning environment.

self-paced programs Instructional programs based upon an individual child's learning style and rate of learning.

sensory integration A therapeutic technique commonly used to modify neurological dysfunctions in children who are cerebral-palsied, learning-disabled or mentally retarded.

service delivery system A full range of special education placement options, from full-time placement in regular education to placement in a 24-hour residential facility.

speech conservation Treatment services delivered to children with *acquired* hearing impairments for purposes of preserving and enhancing speech production skills acquired prior to onset of the hearing impairment.

speechreading A method of teaching a hearing-impaired child to make use of visual cues and other information as an aid in helping to better understand what is being said.

spina bifida A birth defect resulting from the failure of the spinal column to close completely, causing a physical disability.

state education agency (SEA) A state department responsible for the administration of public school education.

stoma care Antiseptic care of the external surgical opening on the body due to a colostomy or an ileostomy.

suctioning Use of equipment to draw out secretions or mucus.

synchrony of movement A smoothly flowing, well-coordinated, and controlled movement of the body and its parts.

talking book A long-playing record used by blind and partially sighted children.

teleteaching Teaching homebound children via a special telephone hook-up.

tube feeding Artificial means of giving nourishment through a tube.

Author Index

Subject Index